66

Weight loss...in a **different light**

"I tried to diet a million times, and a million times I failed. Day after day, Monday after Monday, New Years after New Years I would vow to *start fresh*..." *(page 5)*

"Don't let your body get bored. Bored=stored fat." *(page 81)*

"No one or diet is perfect." *(page 101)*

"Think that's too much? How much time to you spend watching TV? Surfing the web? Talking on the phone?" *(page 145)*

"It's not about the donuts. It's about the person who upset you, or the extra work, or the fatigue, or the hopelessness." *(page 148)*

"What no one really talks about, though, is the main reason many of us fail with our weight loss efforts: our minds won't let us." *(page 147)*

99

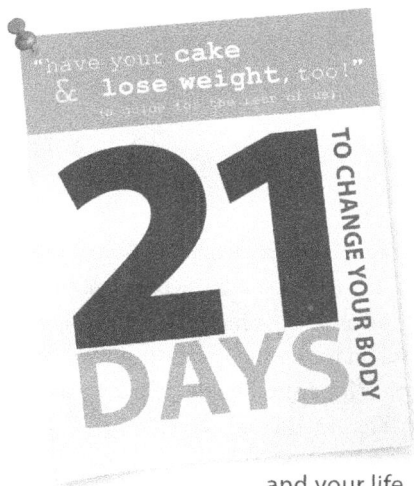

"have your cake
& lose weight, too!"
(a hope for the rest of us)

21

DAYS

TO CHANGE YOUR BODY

...and your life

ignite weight loss

and **start living**

by Helen. M. Ryan

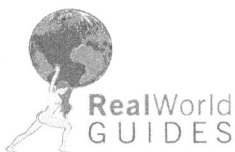

RealWorld
GUIDES

Copyright © 2012 by Helen M. Ryan

Published by Real World Guides

ISBN-13: 978-0615641911
ISBN-10: 0615641911

Book Website
www.21daystochangeyourbody.com

Publisher Website
www.realworldguides.com

Printed in U.S.A

To the loves of my life,
Ryan and Kyra,
with whom I gladly share my chocolate

To my muse and sanity-keeper,
AJ Ogaard
Without his support, this book might not
have been completed
(Twitter: @ajogaard)

Special thank you to:
Karen Grove, freelance editor,
for her editing talents.
(www.karengrove.com)
Linda Wunderlich
for the final look-over

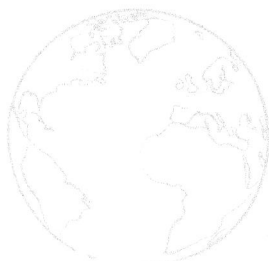

Contents

The Days

Resources

The End

...Is the Beginning

" Every moment is a fresh beginning."

~ T . S. Eliot

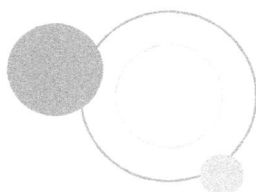

In the End...

*I decided to put the end at the beginning, because—
as with your body—we need to shake things up.*

I could have written a book on super quick weight loss with
impossible and dangerous tricks and made tons of money.

I could have sold you the Brooklyn Bridge with promises of
losing 10 pounds a week with no effort on your part.

Dreams sell, you know?

But real life is not about dreams, and I am not about selling
people. I am about helping people do the best that they can
and to be the best that they can—to find a body that works
for them and a life that's fulfilling. One life is all we have.

Not everyone can be a size 2.
Not everyone is willing to work out two hours a day.

And why, really, should you? Being super thin will not make
you any happier. Trust me on that one: I have been there.
I was once "fittest in the land" and I was pretty unhappy.

Now, I am super fit, regular weight, and mostly super happy.
Because I have found balance. And peace.

Introduction

TOMORROW NEVER COMES

"Tomorrow is often the
busiest day of the week."

~Spanish Proverb

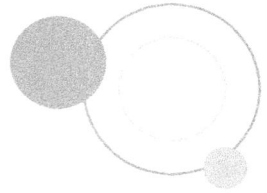

Tomorrow Never Comes

Once upon a time, in the not too distant past, I stood 5 feet tall, weighed 198 pounds and wore a size 20. I could not walk very far, I could not climb stairs, and my body hurt all the time. I was unhealthy and going nowhere, fast.

What saved me was death—and a life-changing experience.

This life-changing experience was holding my father's hand while he died—and finally facing my own mortality. It made me think of all the things I'd never done while waiting for another "tomorrow." Waiting for the day when I'd miraculously wake up thin and fit, with no effort or sacrifice on my part. Waiting for the day when all my dreams would come true—the day when things would finally be different.

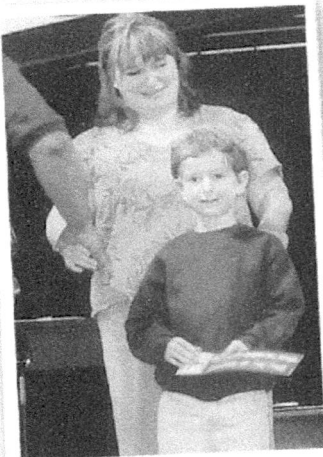

I had spent years waiting, staring into the bottoms of empty ice cream containers, spoon in hand, wondering what had happened to me and my life. Where did I go? Who was this fat, unhappy creature eating away her days, passing time, waiting until she died? I had no answers. The young, fit, happy, passionate,

Waiting for Tomorrow

4

hopeful 20-year-old I once knew was gone. She had been replaced by a sad, overweight, dispirited, hopeless 37-year-old—one who could not even reach her feet to tie her shoelaces. One who was too fat to fit into a ride at Legoland.

I spent my days taking care of children, cleaning the house, running an unfulfilling business, and struggling in a bad marriage. I ate to fill the hole inside and stuffed away the pain with as much junk food as I could. I love my children dearly and would never trade them for anything in the world, but being trapped in a miserable relationship, where nothing seemed to be good enough, had left me empty and void. So I ate. And ate. And ate.

I tried to diet a million times, and a million times I failed. Day after day, Monday after Monday, New Years after New Years I would vow to "start fresh," and this time, darn it, I would succeed. But that success didn't come, so I continued to wait.

Death stopped my waiting.

I never dreamed I would end up losing as much as I did—I just wanted to feel better. I wanted to have less pain, to not have people look at me in pity. "Poor fat girl. No self-control." I used to be strong and healthy. I needed to feel that way again. I needed to show my children that exercise is good, and that our bodies are meant to move. To show them that it feels great to work and stretch your muscles, and that it builds you from the inside, providing mental strength and fortitude, purpose and passion.

I started small by walking the kids to school and back every day. Then I got up early before they rose and exercised in my living room, trying to squeeze exercise in without compromising too much time with my family (and I'm not a morning person). I gave up television completely so I could start taking Spinning® classes (indoor cycling) 2-3 times a week. I changed my eating habits by adding fruits, vegetables, and whole grains to my pitiful, junk food diet, and scoured every health and fitness resource I could find.

I fought hard for my health, but winning the "fat battle" created another problem, because I had finally started fighting for something I'd never championed before: me. I was finally standing up for myself and developing a backbone.

Improving my health ultimately resulted in divorce, but it also gave me new purpose and meaning: to help others by becoming a personal trainer, Spinning instructor, and writer. I could finally contribute something to the world and give positive energy back.

" Less than one year later I was 82 pounds lighter ...and a size 4. "

Now my life is different and mostly good. I have challenges like everyone else, and have good days and bad days. I even put on 15 pounds during the stress of the divorce (but 15 pounds is a drop in the bucket compared to the over 82 that I originally lost).

I raise my children in a positive and healthy environment, even training my son (who is now finally talking to me again after some tough workouts, he, he), and taking Zumba® Fitness classes with my daughter. We have lots of fun, laugh a lot, and they put up with my constant talk of fitness, health and, of course, Spinning.

My new lease on health and life also gave me another unexpected benefit. I returned to my writing roots (even writing for national magazines and web sites); I shoot photographs at rock concerts and interview rock stars. I have ridden hundreds of miles on my bike (including a Century and four times up a mountain), started a publishing company and a nonprofit organization, and designed a line of fitness shirts (see one on page 193). And yet I am a just another average woman over 40—a single, solely self-supporting mother of two.

My goal with this book? To show you what I have learned. To show you that change is, indeed, possible. You don't have to be stuck in your body, and you don't have to be unhappy or unhealthy. Sure we can only change certain things in life (and we can only change things, not people), but we can create our own happiness, and have a moment here and there of joy. We truly are in charge of our own destinies.

The ability to change is in your hands, and I want to show you how to get started. I can't do it for you, but I can lead the way.

It takes 21 days to create new habits, so stop waiting for tomorrow. Start...right now.

Are you with me?

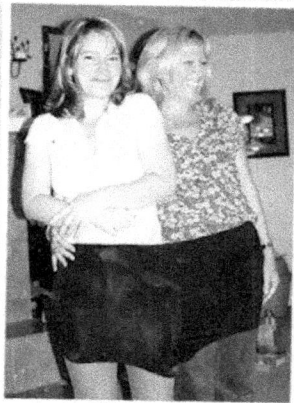

My Old Swim Trunks

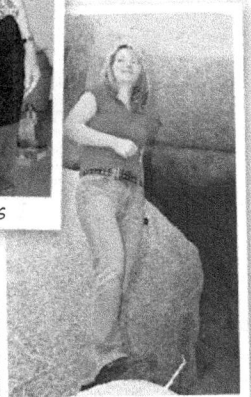

Year 1 – Rebirth

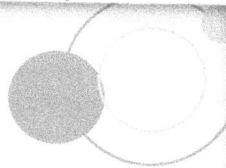

7

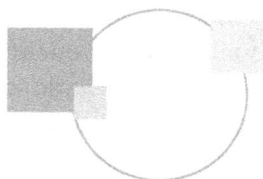

It's Never Too Late

"Maybe we'll turn it around 'cause it's not too late. It's never too late."
~ Three Days Grace

There's nothing easier than losing weight. There's also nothing harder.

The easy part is diet and exercise. We all pretty much know how to eat healthy and we also know that we should be exercising regularly. Weight loss (with a few exceptions) truly is about calories in versus calories out.

We sit a big chunk of our day in cars, offices, in front of our televisions and at our computers. We eat things that are high in calories because "one chocolate bar won't hurt."

We are sometimes _____ (insert: tired, unhappy, sad, stressed, lonely, discouraged, frustrated, angry, fed up) and to quell those feelings, some of us turn to food. Others of us just simply like to eat.

Food is a complicated relationship because we have to eat to survive. For those of us in an "unhealthy food relationship," the daily battle of "don't eat this" becomes too much to handle. So we go ahead and eat the food anyway, believing we will start fresh tomorrow. I know all about this. Believe me—I've been there hundreds, if not thousands, of times.

This book is aimed to help you learn a little more about yourself, think before you eat, make healthier choices and most of all succeed with weight loss.

MAKE ONE CHANGE AT A TIME

Too many changes all at once are hard to keep up with. There is so much to keep track of that you can't focus, and may end up failing once again. Making a bunch of changes at a time is sort of like multi-tasking: you cut back on carbs over here, remove sugar over there, stop drinking coffee, eat more fiber, consume more vegetables, exercise twice a day until you collapse, and pretty soon you are totally burned out, overwhelmed and have gone back to your old habits.

" Weight loss is a sum of all your habits— not individual ones. "

This book is broken down into 21 days for that reason, with 21 fresh, new habits you can follow. In all reality, it would be best to adopt just one of these new habits a week (taking 21 weeks to finish the book). However, I know we are all in a hurry for results, and are accustomed to instant gratification. So take it at whatever speed you'd like. If you find yourself slipping, however, go back to Day 1 and start again, this time focusing on one day for a full week. It took a lifetime to establish bad habits—it will take a little time to establish new ones.

Making gradual changes is very effective and you will reap the rewards. Small changes made every day really do add up. I know it's hard to be patient and wait—I am guilty of that as well. But unless you are extraordinarily driven and disciplined, making a lot of changes immediately won't work. That is the truth. Take it one step at a time.

Crash dieting and crash exercising hasn't worked for you in the past, has it?

Within these pages you will find:

- A quick start guide
- A day-by-day guide to change your mindset and your eating/exercise habits
- Motivational articles (and not the hokey ones—these are things you can probably relate to)
- Bonus weight loss diary excerpt. My true, and funny, struggle to lose the 15 pounds I regained later.

So delve in. Be patient. And if at first you don't succeed, try, try again. Don't give up.

DISCLAIMER

The requisite disclaimer:

I am not a nutritionist. I am not a doctor. I am not a psychologist. I am a woman (and personal trainer) who finally, after years of struggling, lost 82 pounds – and kept most of it off. My battles are the same as yours (and my clients). I share with you what worked, what didn't and what you need to do to lose weight.

In other words, this is real life weight loss. No mumbo jumbo. No "off limit foods." I say it as it is, as it works, and give you choices.

Within these pages you will find some "warm and fuzzy parts" and some "in your face" parts...because sometimes you need both a little handholding and a little push. Also, I have used the word "fat" several places in this book. To me, fat is not a bad word, it's what my kids used to call a describing word. No need for bunching panties. It's time for you to move on with your life, come what may.

If you need the advice of a Registered Dietician (advised in many cases to get you started—especially if you have any medical conditions), visit www.eatright.org. They will help you find a nutrition professional.

P.S. Because music is so important to me and many others, the "Head" chapters use song titles in the headlines. Do you know what songs these are? Or who sings them? Visit my blog www.realworldweightloss.com to see if you're right!

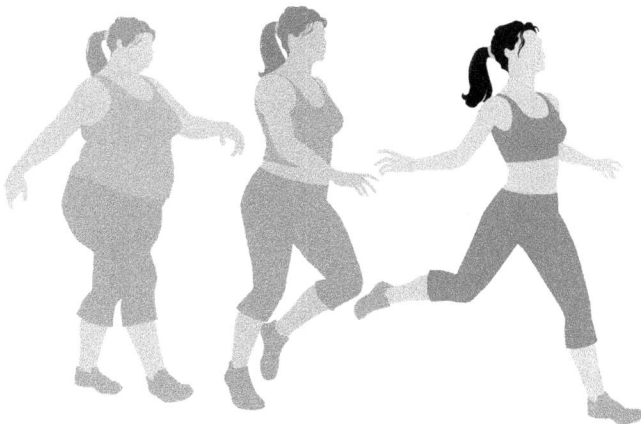

INTRODUCTION

FAQS

Q: Can you lose weight in 21 days?
A: Yup. But a zillion pounds? Nope.

Q: Then why should I read this book?
A: Because in 21 days I will help you to change your mindset, which in turn will change your body.

It takes 21 days to start a new habit. What, really, is a habit? According to the dictionary, a habit is " an acquired behavior pattern regularly followed until it has become almost involuntary." And that is what we are striving for...helping you set a new pattern of healthier behavior that are almost involuntary. That's how thin people live.

Each day is broken down into two sections to make it more manageable: the *Head* section and the *Body* section. For example, Day 1(A) is the "mind" portion (that is where we discuss the mental obstacles to losing weight). Day 1(B) is the "body" portion where you discover specific weight loss tips.

As I said above, weight loss is both easy and hard. It's easy because the rules are fairly simple. It's hard because sometimes the rules don't apply and we have to get creative.

Are you ready? Let's go.

Day 1 is dawning.

Quick Start

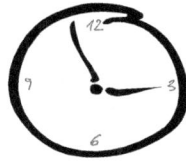

We all want a quick start to weight loss. Even though gaining weight took a long time, we want to lose it *fast.*

Though this book is meant to be read over weeks and use baby steps to help you succeed, there are ways to get the scale to start moving—*quickly.*

Remember, the below tips are not a lifestyle change. These are merely options to get you started with quicker results. A lifestyle change doesn't involve cutting out a certain food or overdoing exercise. Lifestyle changes are about balance—and the ability to lose weight while being happy. But sometimes... you want "quick as a bunny." So here you go:

- Drink a full glass of water before each and every meal.
- Cut out all refined carbohydrates (cookies, cakes, "white" breads and pastas, rice, etc.).
- Eliminate sugars (check labels—hidden sugars are everywhere).
- Limit your carbohydrates (other than vegetables/ fruits) to once per day, or eat less than 25 grams of carbs per meal.
- Increase your lean protein intake. Eat a good 30 grams of protein per meal (with some at snack time) and always start your morning with protein.
- Exercise throughout the day. Schedule a very hard aerobic workout, a hard and heavy brief strength

training session, and every couple of hours, find a way to move. Do squats, step ups, lunges, walk up stairs briskly, jump*...anything that gets you moving and breathing hard for 2-3 minutes. Set your timer (or an online timer) to get you up and out of your chair. Do something at every commercial break. Move, move, move.

- Cut your meals in half (but make sure you don't go too low with the calories or you won't have energy to exercise). Eat half of your usual lunch and dinner sizes, saving your full meal for breakfast.
- Fill half of your plate with vegetables at lunch and dinner and eat those first.
- Brush your teeth after every meal and snack (to get rid of the food taste and keep you from continuing to eat. You will see this tip many times throughout the book. The reason? It works. Incredibly well.)

Use the tools you have...and share you story and journey with me on my blog or Facebook page.

*See page 104 for illustrations/descriptions of exercises.

Book web site: www. 21daystochangeyourbody.com
Blog: www.realworldweightloss.com
Facebook: realworldweightloss
Twitter: aspinchick

DAY
1

"I tried every diet in the book.
I tried some that weren't in the
book. I tried eating the book. It
tasted better than most of the diets."

~ Dolly Parton

DAY 1

YOUR HEAD

A New Body:
Don't You Want Me, Baby?

"All know the way; few actually walk it."
~ Bodhidharma

Yes, we all know the way. Most of us have been bombarded for so long with weight loss information that we do, in fact, know how to lose weight.

Then why don't we?

- Because we are not ready
- We are not willing
- And we don't really want to

I know you think you really want to. But do you truly?

Think back to other things in life you really wanted. The vacation, the car, the concert tickets, the college degree. You worked hard for it, saved and sacrificed. Nothing could stand in your way. You wanted it so badly you could taste it and would do anything to get it.

Now examine your approach to losing weight and becoming healthier.

When was the last time you got up at 5:30 a.m. to fit in some exercise, even if you went to bed late? But would you even question getting up at 3 a.m. to catch a plane to Maui? Losing weight is about shifting priorities. When I finally began seriously losing weight, it was because I had changed my priorities. This change didn't affect my family or work, but it did affect my life overall. I got up early to exercise, even on weekends. I walked the kids to school instead of taking the easy way out and driving. My health became a priority.

When was the last time you put your own health first?

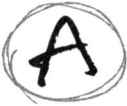

Take Action:
QUESTIONS TO ASK YOURSELF

- **What is holding you back from your goals?**
  (You. But why?)

- **What are your fears?**
  (Your spouse might get jealous? It's a real possibility. How will you handle it?)

- **What are you missing?**
  (Sleep, intimacy, communication, comfort? How can you meet those needs with something other than food?)

- **What does eating those chips, fries, and chocolate actually do for you?** (Other than giving you a momentary good feeling—and it really is a good feeling.)

DAY 1

YOUR BODY

Food, Food Everywhere – A Guide To Eating

A few years ago, while chatting with a friend of mine about weight loss, I mentioned that he should be eating more fiber. This man, who is very intelligent and in his mid-30s, asked me a question that blew me away: "*What's fiber?*"

With that in mind, this chapter helps you get started on a path to healthier eating. I have provided links to many helpful tools in the Resources section of this book (see page 138), from calorie calculators and online food diaries, to reputable weight loss sources where you can get the latest, and greatest, in healthy nutrition news (no fads, there).

CALORIES

Calories are simply energy, but in different forms. You have energy IN (calories in the form of the foods you are eating) and energy OUT (calories in the form of energy you are using).

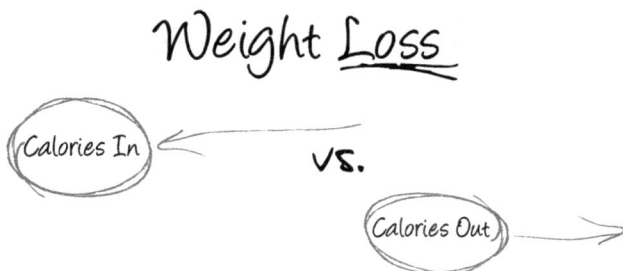

Weight Loss

Calories In ⟵ vs. Calories Out ⟶

Without going into greater detail (or arguing the point of "diet experts" who have created all types of fancy, restrictive diets to sell to you), losing weight is basically calories in versus calories out. When you eat more calories than you use, the "unused" calories are all stored as fat, causing you to gain weight. For weight loss, you need to use more calories than you take in (eat). Your body will then find other energy sources to pull from, like stored fat (and some protein from your muscles—hence the importance of strength training. See page 57).

THE **DAYS**

Calories come in many different forms. I have included a breakdown of the main nutrients, their sources, and generally recognized recommended amounts in the Resources section, page 136 (skip on over there now and take a peek. The more you know, the easier it will be.)

CONTENT & TIMING

Keep in mind that anything you eat in excess that is not used by your body—even the beloved protein—will be stored in your fat cells. Calorie control is truly king, and though weight loss is in simple terms about calories in versus calories out, the way your body uses different nutrients can affect your results.

> Remember— when you exercise, you need food and nutrients. Don't eat so little that you have no energy for working out.

Experiment with different food percentages and diet types to see what works for you. Some bodies respond to a lower carbohydrate diet, some bodies respond to a low glycemic index diet, some bodies respond to a balanced 40-30-30 diet (40% carbohydrates, 30% fats, 30% proteins).

Play around with the time you eat certain kinds of foods, too. For some people, eating a majority of their carbohydrates earlier in the day, or before or immediately after workouts, seems to work best. For others, timing is not really an issue.

SHOPPING

When you are grocery shopping, think of eating as few "man-made" foods as possible and shop mostly around the perimeter of the store. Focus on fresh vegetables, lean meats or vegetable proteins, eggs, and low-fat dairy. Sprinkle in some fruits, and eat very few processed foods. Check labels—if you can't pronounce many of the ingredients in a product, put it back on the shelf.

Most of all: don't confuse low calorie or low fat with health. Jellybeans may be fat-free, but the tremendous jolt of sugar they provide is *not* healthy.

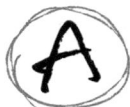

(A) Take Action:

Start reading labels to discover what exactly is in the foods you eat. Pay attention to serving sizes to make better choices. If there is very little nutritional value in the food, pick something else that's similar but packs a better nutritional punch. It's all about giving your body the right foods to do what you ask of it.

DAY
2

"The older you get, the tougher
it is to lose weight because by then,
your body and your fat are really
good friends..."

~ Anonymous

DAY 2

YOUR HEAD

Stop Waiting:
The Joke Is On Me

"Sometimes I can hear my bones straining under the weight of all the lives I'm not living."
Jonathan Safran Foer

Most of us can hear our bones strain from promises unfulfilled. When we spend too much time remembering the past, living for the future, and surviving on daydreams rather than reality, we fail to live for today.

> " We let life live us instead of
> us living our lives. "

We take no action, make no changes, and wonder why we feel empty. Some of us eat to compensate for that emptiness, instead of actually doing something about it.

How many years did I tell myself, *"I'll go to the beach next year when I am thinner?"* I never went (because I wasn't thinner).

How many times did I dream of the things I would do when I got thinner? I didn't do them (because I wasn't thinner).

How much of my life did I let pass by? At least 15 years. One day I was in my early 20s, the next, or so it seemed, I was pushing 40.

Where had those years gone? What had I done with my time, my life, my dreams? Why had I not taken action? I did not know. *Do you?*

Go take a good, long look in the mirror. Then ask yourself the following, out loud (yes, you will feel dumb, but do it anyway).

1) Do I take myself seriously?
2) Do I take my health seriously?
3) Do I treat my life and health as a joke?

Every time you eat something that's not healthy, ask yourself: *"Am I treating myself like a joke?"*

Every time you skip an exercise opportunity (even if it's just a 10-minute walk or a game of tag with your kids), ask yourself again: *"Am I treating myself like a joke?"*

We have only one life—we need to start taking it seriously.

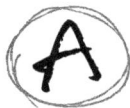

Take Action:

Imagine yourself at 90 years old, looking back on your life. Did you have regrets for the things you did *not* do? For the opportunities wasted because you felt "too fat?" Were there no pictures of you in photo albums? Write down your answers to these questions in a notebook (along with other questions, answers and thoughts you discover along the way) and re-read them frequently.

DAY 2
The Mystical Potion for Weight Loss Triumph

YOUR BODY

Is there a mystical potion when it comes to good health and happiness? There is, indeed.

This mystical potion:

- Helps you lose weight
- Helps you sleep better
- Puts some oomph back into your sex life
- Reverses the negative effects of stress
- Improves learning and memory
- Makes you happier and less depressed
- Helps you live longer
- Improves your health by lowering bad cholesterol, increasing good cholesterol; prevents and controls diabetes; lowers your blood pressure; reduces risk of stroke; decreases risk of osteoporosis; strengthens your heart and lungs
- Reduces PMS symptoms and lessens mentrual cramps
- Gives you more energy
- Helps your posture and reduces back pain
- Lubricates your joints and builds muscle

...and a ton of other benefits too long to list.

What is this magic and why haven't you heard of it before? You have. It's called *exercise*.

Only two out of 10 Americans get the recommended amount of exercise. Why? Probably because they hate it.

Exercise doesn't have to be hateful, but in all reality, nothing else does for your body what exercise does. Even if you consider it a chore, aren't there plenty of other things you don't like to do that you do anyway? And those aren't as good for you as exercise.

If exercise truly is this magical, why wouldn't you do it?

A design client recently asked me, after I had finished a long and grueling deadline, how I could head off to the gym to teach a Spinning class when I was so exhausted. My answer: because I have to, for my health and peace of mind. Sometimes I would rather shoot myself in the face than get on that bike. But I go, anyway. It's part of my life now, it's who I am, it keeps me healthy, and it helps me stay moving ahead with my life. I truly believe that without regular exercise, I couldn't do all the things that I do. I would have neither the stamina nor the mental strength to forge forward.

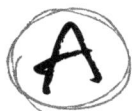

Take Action:

List your own reasons to exercise (by priority). List the excuses why you do not. Compare the two. Sure, you don't have much time in your day, but as the old saying goes, *"Would you rather exercise one hour a day or be dead 24 hours a day?"* Now, get out there and do something. Right now. Even if only for 10 minutes. **Go.**

EXERCISE

Want to **sleep better**?

Put some **passion** back into
your **sex life**?

Be **smarter**?

Feel **happier**?

Live **looooonger**?

Reduce **PMS** symptoms

Get more **energy**?

Reduce your back pain?

Lose weight?

Then...
EXERCISE!

DAY
3

"The only place where
success comes before work
is in the dictionary."

~ Vidal Sassoon

DAY 3
YOUR HEAD

The Magic Bullet: Dirty Little Secret

"This is the world we live in. And these are the hands we're given...."
~ Genesis

There is a magic bullet when it comes to weight loss.

It doesn't cost money, it's not hard to get, and it's not only for a special, select few. In fact, you already possess this magic tool: look down. It's your hands.

> The power to change is in my hands.
>
> Repeat after me.
>
> The power to change is in my hands.

Our hands rub backs, fold laundry, wield hammers, reach out, type, and communicate. Our hands are the magic bullet because they control what we put in our mouths, and they control if we open the door to get out and exercise.

The power to change is in your hands. You have the single most important tool to weight loss right in front of you, and you've had it all along. That tool is you. No one is going to come and rescue you. No one else is going to help you get healthier or thinner. No one else is going to control what you eat, or whether or not you exercise. You are the writer of your own life story.

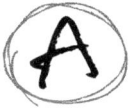

Take Action:

Look at your hands. Turn them over, palms up. Turn them
back around again.

Now, no matter how silly you feel, and you may feel pretty
silly, say the following action phrase: *"The power to change
is in my hands."* Say this while you are looking at your hands.
Walk over to the fridge or pantry and pull out something you
like that is not very good for you. Hold it in one hand, and
keep the other one palm up. Again, say the action phrase:
"The power to change is in MY hands." Put the item back
(don't eat it!)

From now on, and for the next 18 days, say the action phrase out
loud (if you can) every morning and every night—without fail.
Don't be shy...just do it.

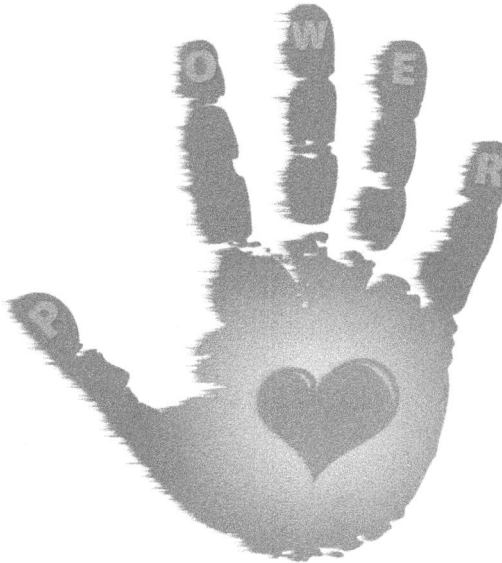

DAY 3

YOUR BODY

How Much Is Too Much? A Portion Size Refresher

Supersize me!

The easiest way to lose weight is to *not* supersize. Portions are grossly oversized, and can be one of the biggest challenges you encounter when it comes to your weight loss.

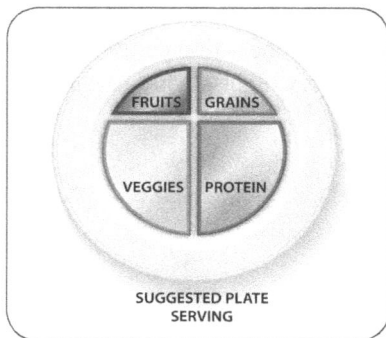

SUGGESTED PLATE SERVING

So how much should you eat? The U.S. Government has done away with the famed food pyramid and has designed the "food plate" instead. Their recommendations? On a 9-inch plate, fill ¼ of it with vegetables, ¼ with fruit, ¼ with lean protein, ¼ with carbohydrates (www. myplate.gov). Some weight loss professionals advocate a slightly modified food plate with ½ veggies, ¼ lean protein, ¼ carbohydrates (and the occasional fruit on the side).

Which works best? Only you know what's a good fit for your body. Try them both for a week each and see how you feel and fare. The dairy? They put it in a cup on the side. I count my own dairy as protein, so I stick it in the protein portion. I'm a major cheese and hot chocolate lover.

Portion Help!

○ **At Home**
  - Use measuring cups and spoons. Remember—measuring only needs to be done in the beginning (at least a few weeks). Once you get the hang of how much a serving really is, you will be better able to tell with just at a glance. (See infographic on serving sizes, next page.)
  - Never eat directly from the original box, bag, or container. Serve it up in a small bowl or onto a small plate. Keeping your hand out of the chip bag cuts down on mindless eating.
  - Choose smaller plates like salad plates and soup-bowls. We're tempted to fill our plates all the way, so using these smaller sizes is a lot better for your waistline.

○ **Dining Out**
  - My favorite trick when eating out is to request a box when my meal arrives and immediately put half of the meal in it. It may feel funny at first, but it definitely helps reduce the temptation to keep eating. If it's in front of us, we'll eat.
  - Order kids' meals. The child menu portions are generally smaller (just skip the fries).

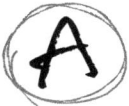

THE DAYS

A Take Action:

Buy a 9" fun kids' plate and use that for your meals. I am very fond of my Scooby Doo plate.

Visual Portion Sizes

Meat (3 oz.) = Deck of cards

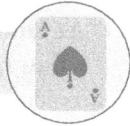

Pancake (1) = CD

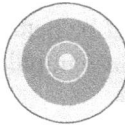

Rice (1 cup) = Tennis ball

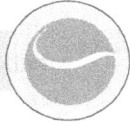

Pasta-cooked (1 cup) = Baseball

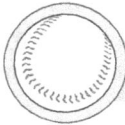

Peanut butter, 1 tbsp = One die

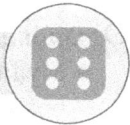

Cheese (1 oz.) = Lipstick tube

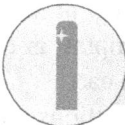

Medium or cut fruit = Lightbulb

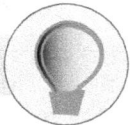

Baked potato = Computer mouse

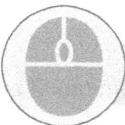

DAY
4

"Inside some of us is a thin
person struggling to get out,
but they can usually be sedated with
a few pieces of chocolate cake."

~ Author Unknown

DAY 4
YOUR HEAD

Devil Inside:
Self-Control

"Self-respect is the root of discipline the sense of dignity grows with the ability to say no to oneself."
~ Abraham Joshua Heschel

Constant self-control can break many a diet. We have to control what we eat, what we drink, what we think, and how much we exercise.

Meal after meal, day after day, we resist temptation. It can seem insurmountable at times. Maybe even impossible. It's not. There is a very bright side to self-control: it gives you freedom and peace of mind. *"How?"* you might ask. By you controlling food and not letting food control you.

Binging is actually a form of control. When something in our lives is out of control, eating may be the only thing we *can* control. While anorexics control their situation by *not eating*, overeaters often control their situation by *eating*. Wresting positive control of yourself is indeed freeing—it's the proverbial monkey off your back.

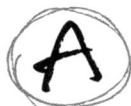

(A) Take Action:

Self-control is truly like a muscle. The more you flex it, the stronger it gets. Give it a workout this week.

How To Get Started With #*!#&!@ Exercise

DAY 4

YOUR BODY

The variety of exercise options out there can be overwhelming, and the many questions can make you crazy. Where do you start? What do you do? How much? How often?

Don't worry. The best fitness program is the one that works for *you* (to see what worked for me, read Day 6). It doesn't matter what anyone else is doing. Find out what fits into your schedule, your life, and that you enjoy. If you don't like it, even just a little bit, you won't do it. Period.

START SMALL

If you're not consistently exercising now, or you haven't exercised in awhile, start small. Walking is a wonderfully underrated exercise, as is swimming, dancing, and working out on an elliptical machine or an indoor bike. The secret is to take small steps, but to be consistent with them.

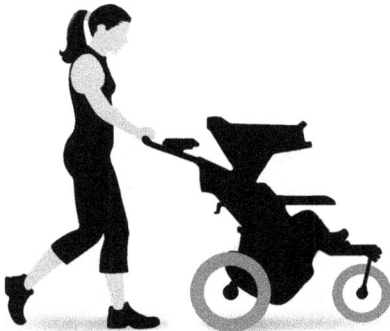

Did I start Spinning classes immediately or curling 15 pounds when I first started? Heck no! I used lighter weights and started walking. That's all my body could do at the time.

THE **DAYS**

35

FIND WHAT YOU LIKE

You may be the kind of person who doesn't like to exercise. But there are the "lesser of two evils", so pick one that works for you. To lose weight, be healthy, and not wind up wheelchair-bound later in life, you have to exercise consistently. There's no way around it.

Sometimes you don't know what you like until you try it, so select a variety of things, making sure to do both strength training and cardio. Danced-based exercise is great fun and a super way to get started with an exercise program. If you don't want to head to the gym, there are many good exercise videos out there you can do in the privacy of your own living room. (I got my start with Tamilee Webb's "*I Want That Body*," working out in my PJs. Thanks Tamilee!). Collage Video has a huge collection of videos, and YouTube has great exercise routines, too. Try different things until something resonates with you. My loves are Spinning, kettlebells, barre, and the TRX® Suspension Trainer™. *What will be yours?*

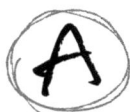

(A) Take Action:

Pick one class this week at your gym that you've never done before and give it a try. Talk to the instructor before class and give him/her a heads-up that you are new. Most instructors love "newbies" and will be more than willing to give you pointers and encouragement. Or head over to YouTube and pick something unique to try: belly dancing, pilates, yoga, bodyweight training...it's all there for you to try. Be different. You might like it.

DAY
5

"I keep trying to lose weight...
but it keeps finding me!"

-Author Unknown

DAY	**Find Your Strength:**
5	**(Nothin' Gonna) Break My Stride**

YOUR HEAD

"You are braver than you believe, stronger than you seem, and smarter than you think."
~ Christopher Robin

We all have unimaginable strengths. They materialize before our eyes in times of crisis. If there is a problem, we step up to the plate and handle it. Questions come later.

So it's time to step up for your own health—to tap into the power that's inside of you. Sometimes the power is straightforward. Sometimes you have to trick yourself to locate it. But the power in gaining control of yourself and your life is at your fingertips and can be harnessed with a few simple tricks:

1. *Never tell yourself "no" when you want a certain food.* Tell yourself "later," instead. If you really want the food later then have it. Right now, though, give yourself some time to get back under control.

   Most cravings last only about 15 minutes or so, then the feeling passes. If you can get through those 15 minutes you are on your way to success. Each time you don't give in immediately to a craving, you become that much stronger—and gain control. Let yourself start to associate the word "no" with something positive.

2. *Realize that some things are beyond your control.* You cannot control other people—what they think and do—but you can control how you feel about it. Take back control of your mind and don't let anyone set up shop in your head. Letting someone make you angry, letting someone put you down, letting someone provoke you puts them in the driver's seat. Don't let them drive. Let it go, and take back your control.

3. *Find something new or slightly challenging to do and push past where you think you can go.* Control your body by giving it just a little nudge. Walk past the point of feeling tired. Lift your weight just a few more times. Finish a project faster than you normally would. Rising to a challenge is a form of control, and the more you do it successfully in your daily life, the easier it becomes with food.

4. *Identify your eating triggers.* Fatigue? Nervousness? Stress? Boredom? Know what they are. When you feel them triggering overeating, go back to item number one and tell them "later."

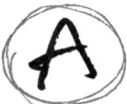

Take Action:

Next time you have a craving, keep yourself busy for about 20 minutes and don't indulge it. Go brush your teeth or use a strong mouthwash to make it less likely you'll eat. If the craving is still there after 20 minutes, find something less damaging to eat. See how far you can stretch your ability to say "*not now.*"

DAY 5 — Breakfast of Champions — The Key to Weight Loss

YOUR BODY

31 million Americans set themselves up for failure every single day.

Why? They don't eat breakfast.

Aside from the fact that you may be cranky after a nightlong fast, not eating breakfast can leave you feeling starved and unable to resist that sugar-filled doughnut at 10 a.m. Skipping breakfast is a surefire way to sabotage your weight loss.

Your mom might have told you breakfast was the most important meal of the day. Guess what? She was right. Here's why you should start your day with fuel:

Breakfast...
- Keeps you from overeating. People who don't eat breakfast tend to eat more later in the day, or snack on higher-calorie foods throughout the day.
- Gives you more energy. Breakfast eaters have more stamina and strength than non-breakfast eaters.
- Helps you think more clearly. A balanced breakfast of a complex carbohydrate with protein will keep your brain on track. (High-sugar cereals? Nix those. Too much sugar actually impairs your thinking.)
- Keeps your appetite down by increasing your levels of the appetite-suppressing hormone leptin.

78% of the 5,000 people in the National Weight Loss Registry—who lost an average of 66 pounds—ate breakfast every day. Why wouldn't you?

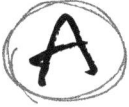

(A) Take Action:

Start each day with a protein-filled breakfast. Protein helps keep you full longer and gives you a good, balanced start to your day. Think one whole-grain slice of bread with a vegetable omelet, or—my favorite—unsweetened oatmeal made with nonfat milk and fat-free cottage cheese on the side. (I also love oatmeal/egg white/protein powder "pancakes".)

THE **DAYS**

Quick Breakfast Ideas

- Protein powder smoothie
- Coffee protein smoothie
- Protein pancakes or protein pancake rollup
- Waffle with peanut butter & cottage cheese
- Fat free plain greek yogurt with trail mix
- Egg/canadian baconwich
- Fat free cottage cheese with berries
- Oatmeal (with milk) and almonds
- Microwave omelette
- Protein bar

(Quick breakfast recipes on next page. And visit my blog at www.realworldweightloss.com for more.)

Quick Breakfast Recipes

- **PROTEIN POWDER SMOOTHIE**
  Milk, almond- or soy milk.
  1 scoop of protein powder
  1 packet stevia
  Frozen unsweetened berries

- **COFFEE PROTEIN SMOOTHIE**
  Same as above, but freeze coffee in an ice
  cube tray, and add coffee ice cubes instead
  of frozen berries.

- **PROTEIN PANCAKES OR
  PROTEIN PANCAKE ROLLUP**
  ⅓ cup rolled oats
  ¼–½ tsp baking powder
  ¼–⅓ scoop vanilla protein powder
  1 packet stevia
  ⅓ cup pure egg whites
  Blend. Cook like regular pancakes.
  Top with a thin layer of nut butter and a dab
  of cottage cheese with berries. (For roll up,
  use less baking powder, making a thin "pancake" that rolls up for eating on-the-go.)

- **EGG/CANADIAN BACONWICH**
  1 egg
  2 slices Canadian bacon or ham
  Reduced fat cheese.
  Cook togther in pan, and place on one slice
  of whole wheat bread or bread thin/bagel.

DAY
6

"I am not a glutton –
I am an explorer of food."

~Erma Bombeck

DAY 6

YOUR HEAD

Why Are You Doing This?
I Want You Bad

"It is not easy to find happiness in ourselves, and it is not possible to find it elsewhere."
  - Agnes Repplier

Ask the mystery 8-ball, *"Will I lose the weight?"* and the answer will be, *"Cannot predict now."* Why can't the all-powerful ball foresee if weight loss is possible? The answer is, *"It depends on your reason."*

If you want to lose weight for appearances only, the mystery ball will come back with, *"Very doubtful"* and you might as well just put this book away. Go back to watching TV and dream of the day you'll wear something skimpy to the beach and be desired by all.

Losing weight so you can look "hot," to please someone else, for revenge, or other looks-related reasons will almost definitely guarantee failure.

Why?

Because appearance-only reasoning is not enough of a motivator to lose weight. You won't have what it takes to make the major changes in your life or the sacrifices you have to endure to get there. What is the main reason to lose weight and become healthier? Because if you don't, you might very well die sooner rather than later, or end up bedridden and in pain. That is a strong motivator.

List for yourself the reasons why you want to lose weight. Be honest. It's OK to say you want to look better as long as you also have some real, tangible health reasons.

THE GOOD, THE BAD AND THE UGLY— REASONS TO LOSE WEIGHT

Put a checkmark next to your reasons to lose weight (other than appearance).

- ☐ **Health.** Does your back hurt? Do you need to lower your cholesterol, control your blood sugar, strengthen your heart, reduce other risk factors? Do you want more energy, clearer thinking, longer-lasting joints?

- ☐ **Living.** Do you want to live life with freedom and not be controlled by food? Do you want to go to a restaurant and not be judged for what you are eating? Do you want to be able to play with your kids, walk your dog, mow your lawn, swim in the ocean?

- ☐ **Memories.** Are there no photos of you because you felt too fat to be in them? No moments captured on film? Is every shot with your children one without you in it because you were ashamed of the way you looked?

- ☐ **Experiences.** Have you done almost nothing that you wanted to? Are you waiting to experience new things until "tomorrow," when you are thinner, and when you have the physical stamina to do them? Is your life empty of new challenges?

☐ **Getting stronger.** Would you like to be able to carry your own groceries, go hiking, bring a sleeping child in from the car, hang Christmas lights, move furniture, or clean a pool on your own?

☐ **Setting examples**. Do you want to set an example for your kids? Teach them about patience, self-control, pride, making healthy choices, taking care of themselves?

My own goal was simple. After struggling for years to lose weight—battling food my entire life—I decided one day to stop dieting and start living. To not be afraid to go to the beach anymore. And until I could wrap my head around losing weight, say, *"Take me or leave me. I am not ashamed."* My one goal was to become fitter, healthier....and happier.

I gave up trying to lose weight. Gave up fighting with food. Packed in the weight loss towel. And then I was suddenly 82 pounds lighter.

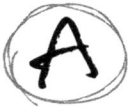

Ⓐ Take Action

Make a list of reasons why you want to do this. Prioritize them and write them down in your notebook. What is most important? What is not? And are these reasons more important than the momentary pleasure that box of cookies or steak brings you?

Movement:
It's an Everyday Thing

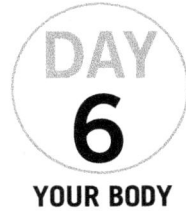

Everything you do burns calories, and burning calories helps you lose weight.

If you are like most Americans, you drive everywhere, exercise rarely, and watch an average of 4.5 hours of television a day. Add to that the time you spend sitting in front of your computer, talking on the phone, or texting, and most of your day is dedicated to...not moving.

The secret to successful weight loss is a combination of eating less and exercising more. If you start only with cutting calories you run the risk of burning off some of your muscle mass and lowering your metabolism.

If you've followed the previous days you are starting to master the eating part. Now—it's time to set your body in motion.

- Do some kind of exercise *every day.*
- Park further away from the store, take the stairs, carry your groceries in one bag at a time, play with your kids, break into dance, squat while you do dishes, mow the lawn, have some sweaty romantic encounters.
- Make it a point to go for at least one 10-minute walk a day (separate it from your harder, regularly-scheduled exercise sessions).
- Break exercise into smaller chunks you do every single day (cardio at one time, strength training at another).

- Get up from your sofa at *every* commercial break and do step ups on your stairs, knee lifts or jumps.
- Set a timer on your computer and break away from your desk every 30 minutes and do same as above. (In fact, I'm doing that right now as I write this.)

What worked for me? I got up super early every morning before the kids woke up and did 15 to 20 minutes of strength training (upper body with dumbbells and pushups one day, then squats, lunges, step ups on a high step stool, planks and crunches the next). Three days a week I walked my kids to school, then later, added Spinning classes 2-4 days a week.

Though my daily schedule would change and fluctuate depending on what crises occurred with small children or business, I could always count on my early morning strength workouts in the dark in front of the morning news.

How much exercise do you really need to lose weight? The American College of Sports Medicine recommends 250 minutes per week to actively lose weight. Want to learn more? Read *"How Much Exercise is Enough to Lose Weight?"* on page 144.

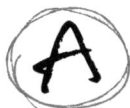

(A) Take Action:

Figure out what you are going to do to move more. Try one new thing each day until you have a whole set of new habits by these next seven days. Remind yourself to follow the guidelines. If you truly want to lose weight, you need to keep moving.

DAY
7

"I'm not overweight. I'm just
nine inches too short."

~Shelley Winters

DAY 7
YOUR HEAD

Change Your Focus:
I Can See Clearly Now

"It isn't that they can't see the solution. It is that they can't see the problem."
-G.K. Chesterton

Once you figure out your main reasons why you want to lose weight (Day 6), start changing your priorities and moving your physical and mental health towards the top of that list.

Also, pick a physical thing you would like to try or excel at and add that your priority list. Selecting a physical goal gives you a real mission and helps you take action. If you want to windsurf, for example, you'll need to strengthen your stomach, back, and legs, and work on your balance. If you want to shoot wildlife photography, aim to increase your stamina and ability to walk distances with a camera pack.

Stop trying to lose weight and shift your focus to doing things that will bring meaning to your life. Being a size smaller is not going to make a big difference in your life unless you are a model. But being healthier and happier definitely will.

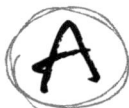

(A) Take Action:

Make a master plan of your priorities, then figure out what you need to do to bring them to life.

Calorie Change-Up: Your Fat Blaster

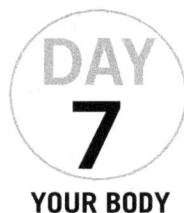

DAY

7

YOUR BODY

Your body likes you to be boring and predictable.

It likes to know you will eat an approximate number of calories a day, and use an approximate number of calories a day. It craves routine and status quo, which keeps it secure in the knowledge that its fat supply is safe.

When you go on a "diet" and eat a set number of calories a day, you can actually help your body keep its fat stores. At first you lose weight because your body is surprised—you are suddenly moving and eating less. A few weeks or months into your program, though, weight loss starts to slow down. To fix this, you might cut back on food even more, but now you're cranky, tired, hungry...and still not losing any more weight.

It's time to shake things up. Calorie cycling to the rescue.

Calorie cycling works amazingly well for both body and mind. It simply means you vary the number of calories you eat each day while still keeping to the approximate total number of calories you need for the week, surprising your body.

The beauty of alternating your calories like this is that it's easier to fit in "cheat days" (if you subscribe to those—see Day 13), or to plan for special events or days where you know you'll be eating a bit more. There's no "blowing it" with this type of eating, which is great for your mind.

THE **DAYS**

51

Varying calories is actually pretty easy. Some days you eat more, some days eat less. For example, on days where I teach Spinning I eat more. On days where my activity is down I eat less. A client of mine, who lost 90 pounds, ate healthy and "clean" most weekdays, and relaxed her eating on weekends (though in the beginning she was stricter).

> Another way to cycle your diet? Change the types of foods you eat. You can, for example, have a caveman day, a vegetarian day, a raw foods day, and so on.

Play with what works for you to find a perfect balance. This is not a license to "pig out," but rather a way to make losing weight fit into your life. We can't control every holiday, wedding, girls' night out, or birthday that comes along. Nor can we hide out at every event, avoiding food.

Whatever you do, just don't be predicable. Make it a game and aim to win.

It's actually sounding kind of fun now, isn't it?

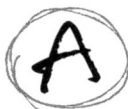

Ⓐ Take Action

Look at your calendar and loosely plan in your calories for the coming week just to get into the swing of things. Pick your "normal," "high," and "low" days (and factor in different types of eating). See how closely you can stick to this—and how it makes you feel. It might take a few weeks to "unstick" your body. Don't get discouraged.

DAY
8

"Rich, fatty foods are like destiny:
they too, shape our ends."

~ Author Unknown

DAY 8

Overpowering the Monster: Fear

YOUR HEAD

"There are very few monsters who warrant the fear we have of them."
    -Andre Gide

FEAR

What keeps many of us from moving forward is our fear: fear of change, fear of hunger, fear of exertion, fear of pain. Fear. The four letter word.

Fear can be paralyzing, but can it keep you fat? Maybe. We can fear hunger. Many of us are not used to feeling hungry, and sometimes being hungry is not so bad as long as there is a meal or a healthy snack on the horizon. Don't lose control at the store because your stomach is growling. Don't eat four bowls of chips at the restaurant because you are "starving". The more occasional "hungries" you overcome, the more in control you will feel.

> " What we should fear is becoming stagnant, and not changing or taking chances. "

Sometimes you should be hungry, like when you wake up in the morning. It's not a crisis. It's hunger, and a bout now and then won't hurt you. If anything, trial runs of hunger will help teach you to gauge when you truly are hungry, rather than eating by the clock. Listen to your body...and learn.

CHANGE

We also fear change. Going from fat to fit is a huge change, so naturally we fear it. As much as we believe we want to weigh less, we fear the unknown. For every action, there is a reaction. We might not be ready for the reaction our new bodies get.

If you feel resistance to losing weight, ask yourself if that resistance is grounded in fears like these:

- **Will your problems be over when you reach your goal?**
  (What if they are not?)

- **Will your significant other feel threatened?**
  (How will you deal with that?)

- **How will you handle attention from others?**
  (Will it make you glad or uneasy?)

- **Will your kids, friends, family think you are selfish?**
  (How will you feel if they do?)

- **How will you find the time to do it all?**
  (And will you go crazy trying?)

Make a list of the fears and cons of losing weight and taking care of yourself. For each question, ask yourself, *"What is the worst that can happen?"*

It might not be as bad as you think. Let go of the fear.

THE DAYS

PAIN

Pain is also a fear we face. Realistically, exercise does involve some pain. Not always, but to see real change there will be some discomfort. Is that necessarily bad? No, because pain makes you stronger. Pain makes you more resilient. Pain builds character. The mental pain of making a choice between an apple and a bag of chips? It's a temporary pain...one that is actually less painful than waking up the next day so full of salt you can't bend your fingers.

Pain is relative and based on your perspective. It's time to change your view of it.

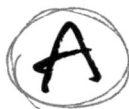

Take Action

Take a walk and think for a moment. Connect with yourself deep down. What are you fears? Are they realistic? Is there anything you can do to see if they're real and valid? And if so, how might you handle them?

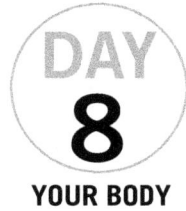

Get Firm:
Cold, Hard Steel

THE **DAYS**

I used to be an avid weight lifter and hated anything cardiovascular. I would run, but hated every minute of it. Sometimes I would ride my bike to school, but only out of necessity because I didn't want to take the bus. For the thrill of it, the power of it, and the invincibility of it I would always lift weights. Nothing beat the feel of cold, hard, heavy steel in my hands.

Now that I've gotten older I have switched teams and am a die-hard cardio fiend (in the form of Spinning and cycling). How and when this traitorous change happened I am not sure. All I know is that I've played on both sides equally, and aerobic exercise is now my drug, I mean exercise, of choice.

However much I like cardio, though, I still strength train. To lose weight, and maintain what you've lost, you need both aerobic exercise and weight training. Strength training gives you a longer calorie burn after exercising, while aerobic activity burns off large amounts of calories instantly.

They really are the yin and yang to each other.

Strength training:
- Gives you a longer "after burn" post-exercise
- Increases your muscles' size and strength (or "tones you up" as some like to say)

- Helps you burn more calories throughout the day since muscles need more calories to just survive
- Increases your bone density
- Helps you look thinner because muscles, while heavier, take up less room than fat

How to do it? There are many ways to strength train, from lifting dumbbells and barbells, to training with body weight and tubing. You can even do it in the privacy of your own home without fancy equipment. No matter what you choose, the key is to be consistent and train hard. If you're a woman, you won't bulk up, but you will become strong and toned (though you won't accomplish *that* with a 5-pound weight— you have to lift a bit heavier).

See the Resources section at the back for tips on what to do, how to get started, and how to see dramatic improvements in your body.

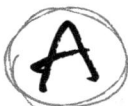

Take Action:

Review the weight training you currently do (if any). Is it too easy? How can you challenge your muscles more? This week, make sure you work your muscles until they are very tired after each workout. You want to feel the accomplishment of a muscle that's fatigued.

DAY
9

"Your body is the baggage you must carry through life. The more excess the baggage, the shorter the trip."

~ Arnold H. Glasgow

DAY 9

All or Nothing: Bad to the Bone

YOUR HEAD

"There is nothing either good or bad, but thinking makes it so."
~William Shakespeare

The biggest saboteur to weight loss success is the 1-0. The on–off. The black–white, all–nothing, good versus bad.

Labeling something bad immediately makes it irresistible (*"bad boy?" "bad food?"*). Every day we make choices between "good" and "bad" food, and how much more fun is bad? If you repeatedly tell a child that alcohol or sex is bad, (all, of course, while indulging in it yourself), do you think they might be tempted to partake in the bad stuff? You bet!

When we differentiate between good and bad foods there is no room for negotiation. Sometimes, just eating a single bite of a "bad" food can lead to uncontrollable binging. If you eat a "bad food," you may feel like you've blown it and now have license to continue the "bad food" eating the rest of the day...and the next day. And the next.

When will a brownie just be a brownie? When you remove the label of "bad" and take away the food's power. But what if foods weren't bad at all? What if *all* foods were really OK if you ate them in moderation? That is what you are going to aim for: it's all OK.

Think about this: one month from now, what will the damage be if you eat one chocolate chip cookie today? Nothing. But one month from now, if that cookie turns into a two-week binge, will there be any damage? Probably about 3-5 pounds worth.

> " I'll say the magic words again:
> take away the food's power. "

Yes, it's delicious and wonderful and makes the chemicals in your brain jump for joy, but it's just food. Eat half the cookie. Brush your teeth. Save the other half for tomorrow.

It's just food.

Don't let it win.

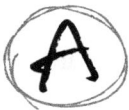

Ⓐ Take Action

Be strong. Take a few bites of your favorite food or snack. Then put it down, go brush your teeth, and move on with your day. Did this bite lead to eating more of it or similar foods? If it didn't, you are on your way to moving forward. If it did, stop, think, and try again another day. It's never too late to be successful. One day you *will* make it.

DAY 9

Starving Yourself...
Fat

YOUR BODY

Do you believe going hungry makes you thinner?

Think again.

Skipping meals in order to lose weight, or look thinner, is a big mistake. I'm not saying that going to bed every now and then a little hungry is a bad thing—it gets you ready for breakfast, teaches you that a bit of hunger isn't always bad, and helps you feel somewhat empowered. But regularly skipping entire meals is a really bad idea. Here's why.

Eating at regular intervals:
- Keeps your blood sugar stable, which powers your brain
- Lets your body run full steam ahead
- Helps prevent diabetes and may even decrease your risk of heart disease

Keeping your sugars sailing smoothly also puts you in a better mood, as the people around me will tell you.

The best way to keep your blood sugar on even keel is to eat every few hours. Plan three meals and three healthy snacks, and make sure the meals or snacks are not just a simple carbohydrate ("white" products such as bread, pasta, rice, cookies, pastries, etc.). Even snacks designed for specific weight loss programs can be loaded with sugars, which in turn will upset your body's balance. A spoon of peanut butter, low-fat string cheese, a small handful of nuts, or a hardboiled egg are all excellent ways to keep your blood sugar stable. A slice of reduced-fat coffee cake? Not so much.

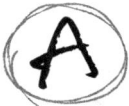

Take Action

Make sure you have healthy snacks in the house that will keep your blood sugars stable. If you do eat a more simple carbohydrate (crackers, for instance), pair it with some low-fat cheese. Remember, though, that not everyone needs to snack. Some people feel better just eating three meals a day. So if it doesn't work for your body—don't do it. Always do what makes you feel the best, strongest, and healthiest.

hardboiled eggs light cheese

lean meats *plain yogurt* nuts

cottage cheese

veggies peanut butter

DAY
10

"The trouble with jogging is that, by
the time you realize you're not in
shape for it, it's too far to walk back."

~Franklin P Jones

DAY 10

Had, Have, Will Have: Time In a Bottle

YOUR HEAD

"Time is a dressmaker specializing in alterations."
~Faith Baldwin

Staying on track with healthy eating and exercise habits is difficult when you feel deprived or sense that you are missing out on something. Saying "no" most of the time to unhealthy choices is not easy. But as you start feeling challenged, just stop for a minute and think about all the *yes's* you did have... the times you ate whatever you wanted, when you wanted (which is how most of us got fat in the first place).

> " Take a look at your past. Eating all that food and not exercising was pretty fun, wasn't it? You had some good times. "

Now look at the present. It's time to crack down and pay the piper. There is no such thing as a free lunch, so start by eating healthily 90% of the time, with a 10% "margin for error" (or "margin for fun.") When you have lost the weight, you can move to an 80% healthy/20% fun plan. Sacrifice now for a huge payoff tomorrow.

The future is about learning balance; to balance mostly good eating with an occasional indulgence, and to get enough exercise to keep you healthy and at the weight you want to be.

You have to work harder now—in the present—to lose the weight and get in shape. It took you years to get fat and out of shape. And yes, you will still have to work to maintain your new weight in the future. Maintaining is not as difficult as losing fat and gaining strength and endurance, though.

Balance.

The past was fun. The present is hard. The future will be exciting.

Remember: it's not this challenging forever. But the health benefits you will reap will last a lifetime.

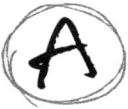

Take Action

What you did in your past caused your present. What you do in your present creates your future. Every action today has a reaction in tomorrow. Think for a moment before you compromise your future health for a momentary pleasure today.

DAY 10 — Sweat...It Does Your Body Good

YOUR BODY

I'm not going to lie.

Spinning hard and strong makes me very happy. My thighs are pumping, my heart is beating fast, and I am doing more than glowing—I am dripping, soaking, utterly wet. What makes me happy, mostly, is that I am under the influence of a drug that is perfectly legal, cheap, and very potent: endorphins.

Endorphins are the "happy" chemical you release during hard exercise. You may know it as "runner's high," but it's all the same.

> " I call it 'chasing endorphins,' and I chase them with challenging aerobic exercise. "

Cardiovascular exercise is the other half of the weight loss equation. As I mentioned on page 57, it's the yin to the yang of strength training.

Aerobic exercise:
- Burns a lot of calories right off the bat
- Helps you become leaner overall
- Increases your lung and heart size and function
- Releases endorphins (the pain-killing chemicals)
- Puts you in a better mood
- Circulates fresh oxygen throughout your body (and helps you feel more alert)

What you choose do to for cardio is up to you. Run, walk briskly, cycle outdoors or indoors, dance, hula hoop, ski, do plyometrics, step, use indoor cardio equipment, play tennis or racquetball — your choices are endless. The trick is to find something you'll actually do, and stick with.

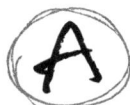

(A) Take Action

Try a new aerobic activity every week until you find a couple that you really like. Make sure you change it up every now and then (even if it's just the length and intensity). If you are working out on cardio equipment at the gym you can alternate with 15 minutes on each of two machines to keep from getting bored.

If you can read a magazine or text while doing your cardio, it's far too easy and you won't see results. You get out of it what you put into it.

THE **DAYS**

BURN CALORIES
SWEAT
ENDORPHINS
FEEL HAPPY
BE FREE&CALM
MUSCLES
GET LEAN
STRONG
HEALTHY
PASSIONATE
CARDIO

"If it weren't for the fact that the TV set and the refrigerator are so far apart, some of us wouldn't get any exercise at all."

~ Joey Adams

DAY 11

Your Comfort Zone: I Want To Break Free

YOUR HEAD

"We think fast food is equivalent to pornography, nutritionally speaking."
~Steve Elbert

Food is an important part of most cultures. People gather around food for birthdays, holidays, and funerals. Friends get together for lunches, and families finally find time to connect with each other over dinner. It is no wonder people associate food with comfort and turn to it when things are not as they should be.

> Find a healthier "comfort food" that still makes you feel good.

Comfort foods are foods that make you happy, that make you feel warm and fuzzy, and that give you a (brief) sense of relief. Sometimes after a long day you can at last sit down, put your feet up...and snack. Finally you are doing something for you.

Breaking the association between food and comfort is difficult, but it's the only way to seriously get on track with weight loss.

Changing a comfort eating habit takes time, awareness, and persistence. It's easy for people to say, "Just fill the 'food void' with something else," but it's not so simple. You'd have to find some other way to relieve stress, soothe nerves, take the edge off sadness, ease loneliness, and help you feel loved. That's a tall order.

When you feel the need to eat, take a few minutes to jot down your moods. Are you:

tired? **stressed?** SAD?

BORED? *happy?*

Next to the emotion, write down what you could do, other than eat, to help get you over the hump. For example, when I am exhausted and have been working at my desk all day I often just want to lay down, put my feet up, and eat some cookies. Instead, I whip out my hula hoop, put on some guilty-pleasure dance music, and hoop for 10 minutes or so. Instant stress relief, re-energizer, and mental boost.

Try playing uplifting music when you are sad, or eating an apple, drinking green tea, or going for a short walk when you are fatigued.

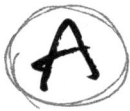

Take Action

Try different things and find what works for you. Everyone is different, and what relaxes others may not work for you. Just be careful not to overcompensate and start habits that are even more detrimental than overeating, like abusing alcohol or other drugs. It's really easy to do.

THE **DAYS**

DAY 11

You Gotta Love It — Eat Foods You Like

YOUR BODY

Whether it was the bad boy in high school or the song we weren't allowed to listen to, the more we were told to not do something, the more we wanted to do it. The same holds true with weight loss. The more you are not supposed to eat that cookie, the more you will focus on it, want it, crave it, think about it, *until you finally break down and eat it.*

> " That's why diets that ban certain foods forever do not work. "

Working things you love into your everyday life is an easier way to stick with your permanent weight loss goals. Short term, it's perfectly OK to cut back, or eliminate, certain foods, as long as you know it's not going to be forever. In fact, if you really want to lose weight, you probably should not be having cookies or wine at all.

However, in the long term an occasional cookie or glass of wine won't kill you or derail your weight loss. While it's good to be stricter in the beginning until you can get yourself under control and your head wrapped around the fact that a chip is just a chip, working a few of your favorites into your daily food choices may help remove the power food has over you—and make your lifestyle diet more sustainable in the long run.

Cutting back on high-calorie, less healthy foods is necessary for quicker weight loss. In order to stick with your program, remind yourself that:

- No food is "forbidden"
- If you truly want it, you can have it tomorrow
- Food is just gasoline for your body—not the meaning of life

If, after reviewing the above, you truly do want the food or drink you are eyeing, then by all means have some—but just a bit. Sometimes, giving yourself a little something will help ward off a full-blown binge.

Once you feel comfortable that you can have just a small amount of your food weakness without losing control, or your weight is closer to your goal, work a favorite into your diet. My favorite? Chocolate. I decided that dark chocolate is a healthier choice than milk chocolate and probably also gives me more "cocoa bang" for my buck. So I incorporate it here and there (including in protein pancakes and oatmeal. Really, how can a day that starts with chocolate be a bad day?)

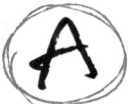

Take Action:

Pick a favorite food that you "can't live without" this week and find creative ways to add a little of it into your diet. Cut the other less healthy foods out and focus on what makes you the happiest. If you love a glass of wine at night after dinner, have your wine, but in a smaller glass. It will be easier to say no to other "play foods" when you know you are giving yourself what you truly, really want.

DAY
12

"I have to exercise in the morning
before my brain figures out
what I'm doing."

~ Marsha Doble

DAY 12

I'm Breaking The Habit... Tonight

YOUR HEAD

"When you are through changing, you are through."
~Bruce Barton

Now that you've established situations in which you tend to use food to provide a temporary fix, it's time to move on to ways you can improve.

Of course, there are a lot of factors involved in getting past comfort eating. Reasons why you feel alone, overwhelmed, empty, stressed, or upset all need to be worked on, but they can't be resolved in this little book. Sometimes, professional help is needed (and there's no shame in that). What I can do here, though, is give you a few tools to start replacing some of the comfort eating you do with other, more productive things—and give you a shot at success.

1. *Exercise really helps.* I know you've heard it before, but it's true. Exercise clears your mind, reduces pain, releases "happy" chemicals, provides a sense of well-being, and reduces stress. If you can find a way to associate exercise with good feelings, you are on your way to solving a big piece of the weight loss puzzle.

   Next time you are really stressed and about to "blow," go outside and take a brisk walk. Or do some angry push-ups. Something that will help you focus on things other than what's upsetting you. Get your heart pumping and move some fresh oxygen through your system. Make it a habit, starting today. Don't respond to that nasty e-mail right now—just walk away and challenge yourself to climb up and down your stairs 20 times. Grab a plastic bat and whack your pillow until you are out of breath. Put the kids in the stroller and go. Dance. Your body was meant to move, so give it what it needs.

Keep trying. Pretty soon you will turn to exercise rather than food for relief.

2. *Find other ways to bring yourself some fulfillment.* Work on a project you have always wanted to do or learn a new skill. Read a "guilty pleasure" book. Again, easier said than done, but at least try.

3. *Treat yourself kindly.* Would you treat someone else the way you treat yourself, placing the same demands on them as you do to your own self, with no rewards or something positive to work toward? I don't think so.

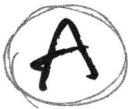

Take Action

Create a "reward system" that does not revolve around food for when you accomplish something. What do you like to do? It might be reading, scrapbooking, writing, making music, photography...anything that gives you a sense of being nurtured or having fun. I know it can't replace your favorite food or snack, but sometimes it just has to be good enough—or you don't move forward.

DAY 12 The Shock! Method

YOUR BODY

We all like a challenge. So does your body.

I know people who do the same exercise routine day in and day out, year in and year out, while complaining that they don't get results. Of course they don't! Curling a 5-pound weight isn't going to challenge your muscle after the first few weeks. Muscles don't grow (i.e. get tighter, stronger, and firmer) without a fight. And your body won't continue to burn fat effectively if all you do is the same cardiovascular workout every time.

" How to add more challenge? Shock your body. "

Shocking your body is a lot like calorie cycling (see Day 7), but with exercise. The same exercise every day will spur your body to become more efficient, and adapt to the physical demands you are placing on it. Once your body adapts, it will burn fewer calories for the same activity.

There are many ways to give your body a wake-up call and trick it into burning more calories and fat. It's just a matter of being creative and not falling into a rut.

Altering your workout is the secret to seeing your body change. Many experts recommend changing your workout every six weeks. I like to change mine (and my clients') workouts every week—and sometimes every session.

For best and quickest results:
- Increase the weight lifted (or the angle, if you are body weight training), or alter the speed and terrain.
- Change the format of the workout with pyramid sets (lighter to heavier), or supersets (two exercises done immediately after one another with no rest in between). Vary your aerobic activity, too.
- Switch up the equipment (alternate between free weights, machines, cables, kettlebells, tubing, suspension training, weighted bars).
- Add stability challenges (exercise balls, unstable surfaces using a single leg, be on your toes, be barefoot, use exercise padding or foam rollers).
- Perform intervals (short, hard efforts followed by a recovery triple the time of the effort) some cardio sessions and steady aerobics (continuous movement at an even tempo) at other times. When working in your interval zone, let your heart fluctuate from mid 60s to the low 90s in percentage. In your consistent zones, keep your heart rate between 70-85% (see Resources page 140 for heart rate tips).
- Change up the amount and type of work you do each week (for example, three strength-training sessions with two cardio sessions one week, and reverse the next week.)

Don't let your body get bored. Bored = stored fat.

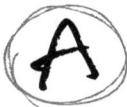

Take Action:

This week, change up the order of your exercises. For example, reverse the order of your strength training circuit, or add hills to your treadmill workout.

THE **DAYS**

"I really don't think I need buns
of steel. I'd be happy with
buns of cinnamon."

~Ellen DeGeneres

DAY 13
YOUR HEAD

Constant Cravings

"We are torn between a craving to know and the despair of having known."
Unknown

Cravings are little weight loss devils. They claw and tear at you, whisper sweet nothings into your ear, and badger you like a peristent 2-year-old until you give in.

Giving in is not necessarily a problem unless eating the food in moderation will spur you to crave more. Sometimes, a handful of chips becomes a bag of chips—and that's where the gremlins lie. The solution? Don't go cold turkey. As soon as you tell yourself "no" you will want it more, so start by cutting back.

If you have a bite, you haven't blown it. Just move on.

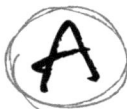

(A) Take Action

Some cravings are brought on by real physical issues. Many women crave chocolate just before their periods. Sometimes thirst will show itself as hunger. Pay attention to your body's cravings. It may be telling you that you need more protein, calcium, fat or sleep.

Cheating...
for a Day

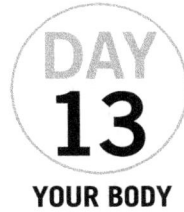

THE **DAYS**

Dieting six days of the week and eating whatever you want on the seventh day? Having a full-on binge-fest and still lose weight? Who wouldn't want that?

The "cheat day" concept became wildly popular when a recent diet book hit the bookstands, though it's been around for ages. The basic idea behind that particular diet's cheat day is similar to calorie cycling, but taken to the extreme and for one day only each week. Scientifically, it is intended to reset the body by giving it a one-day high-carbohydrate break from the "slow carb" diet that lives the other six days.

Cheat day does in many ways have merit, and if you can get it to work into your life—while still losing weight and being healthy—all the better. The biggest problem, other than the health consequences of throwing large amounts of fats and sugars at your body, is that for many of us, once we are "off track" we stay "off track." Cheat day often becomes cheat week, or cheat month or cheat year. Cheat day also reinforces the black-and-white thinking of "bad" versus "good" food, which keeps you chained to "fat" thinking. (Who, really, is ever going to eat tons of broccoli and spinach on cheat day?)

Eating huge quantities of sugar and fat also has another drawback: the food hangover. You know that feeling. You're bloated, puffy, sluggish, tired, constipated, and feel downright miserable. Is your cheat day really worth it?

Options, anyone?

Try a "relaxed day" instead of a cheat day. A relaxed day
is actually very freeing, and it helps remove the good food/
bad food stigma. With relaxed day, you just eat what comes
naturally to you, without forcing a binge or feeling guilty
about what you eat. Want a cookie? Have one. Don't force
yourself to eat the entire box because it's your cheat day.
Nachos? Be my guest. Eat until you start to get full, then
stop. Give yourself permission to eat like a "regular" person,
but not a total pig out. You know as well as I do—when we
eat like pigs, we feel like pigs, and feeling like that is the
worst place we can find ourselves emotionally. We often
already feel bad about ourselves. This kind of feeling won't
help us at all.

You are what you feel, so feel relaxed and at ease with your
food choices. Food is not the enemy.

Something to think about. If you were an alcoholic, would
you abstain from alcohol for six days each week, and then
binge like crazy on the seventh day, drinking a case of beer,
four bottles of wine, and topping it off with a shot of Tequila?

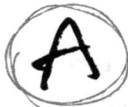

(A) Take Action

Try your first relaxed day and pretend all food is your friend.
Go with your feelings of hunger and eat when you feel like
it. Stop when you're full, stay busy with other things, and
don't think about calories or fat. See if you can go a whole
day eating with a healthy attitude, where food is neither good
nor bad—just necessary. How do you feel after?

"Our bodies are our gardens –
our wills are our gardeners."

~ William Shakespeare

DAY 14

YOUR HEAD

Making Time For You— Priorities

"Take the time to come home to yourself every day."
—Robin Casarjean

If you want to lose weight you have to commit to yourself. There are no exceptions.

Committing to yourself means that you eat what's best for you—not to make others happy. Committing to yourself means mapping out an exercise schedule and sticking to it—come rain or shine. Committing to yourself means you start to put your health needs higher on your list.

When I was actively losing weight I got up early and made exercise a priority. I was sleepy, the house was dark, and I wanted nothing more than to be in my warm, comfortable bed with my "little monsters," as I call them. However, I made my cup of green tea, grabbed a bottle of water, and started pumping (handheld) iron and doing squats before the rest of the house woke up.

If you're not a morning person (and I am not—trust me), you'll have to be a little creative. If anything can go wrong to derail your exercise plans later in the day, it will. Cars break down, kids get sick, shopping needs to be done, deadlines get moved up. But even if it's just 15 minutes, you have to find and make the time. It's your life and health we're talking about.

- Put workouts on your calendar and schedule your appointments around them.

- Make backup plans in case something comes up. Just because you can't make your 6 p.m. step class doesn't mean you can't go for a walk or lunge on your front steps. Missing a scheduled session does not give you free reign to do nothing.

- Fit in whatever you can—make it burn in a good way or elevate your heart rate a bit—and resume your schedule as quickly as possible.

Sometimes it's easier to schedule days A for aerobic activity and days B for strength. That works well for many, as long as you change up your workout in terms of weight, speed, exercise, etc. (see Day 12 – The Shock! Method). Having Mondays-Wednesdays-Fridays be your abdominal and leg day, for example, gives you some structure so if you run out of time you can still plank and squat. Something is always better than nothing. (Did I mention that—perhaps 300 times already?)

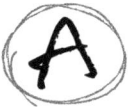

Take Action

Grab a calendar for this week and mark your workouts down in them (if you don't have one, start using one. I live by my Mac's iCal.) Try to maneuver your appointments and commitments around them. Be quiet about it and make it seamless with your life. Pretty soon you'll be seeing big results.

DAY 14 | Stop Dieting: Suddenly I See

YOUR BODY

The best thing you can do for your diet is to stop dieting.

Yup, you read that correctly. On paper, diets sound great and books on the subject fly off shelves. Americans spend $40 *billion* on diet plans each year, and yet we are getting fatter and fatter. Diets in "real life" do not work.

Why?

> " Because the word **diet** makes us immediately think of restriction and sacrifice. Words are incredibly powerful, and **diet** makes us feel uncomfortable, weak, and small. "

You start your diet with the intention of going off of it and returning to your old ways of eating. Looking at the yo-yo dieting many of us have done over the years, with sometimes hundreds of pounds lost and re-gained, we know that this type of thinking doesn't work.

The fix? A lifestyle change. And that's truly what this book is about.

Changing your lifestyle is not as scary or hard as it seems. In fact, it's actually easier than going *on* a diet. The main difference is that you are not forbidding yourself to eat things and you incorporate regular exercise into your life. This sounds easy, right? So why is it so hard?

Lifestyle changes are challenging because they go against everything we've ever been taught. We've been programmed to feel that strict diets are the only way to lose weight, that we have to forever give up our favorite foods, and that we need only to make a change for a short period of time, which technically is far easier to making changes you will do day in and day out for the rest of your life.

Going on a short-term diet leads you to think that you can go back to your chip-eating, beer-drinking, TV-watching life as soon as it's over and you will keep the weight off. If you believe in that kind of magic, you might as well head over to Hogwarts School of Witchcraft and Wizardry. I think Harry Potter's waiting for you.

Back in the real world, we know that losing weight and getting healthy takes sacrifice and commitment. However, lifestyle changes are longer term and often less black and white. Therein lies their beauty. Could you, for a long period of time—long enough to lose some serious weight—give up food such as breads and grains (no pizza, no oatmeal, no nachos, no bagels, no Italian bread, no muffins)? Would you want to? For many of us, I think not. But a lot of us would

Don't Diet Change Your Lifestyle

be willing to cut back short-term and make better choices long-term if we knew that we, indeed, could have these foods in moderation if we truly wanted them.

My favorite way to lose weight is a hybrid method: start out strict, clean up your diet, learn better habits, then slowly begin to work your cleaner eating into a new lifestyle that fits for you. In essence—you start with a healthy "diet" to get your eating on track, learn portion control, educate yourself about different foods and their purposes, reprogram your eating habits and triggers, and then merge that new knowledge with longer-term thinking. A bonus? You'll lose weight faster at the outset, which keeps you more motivated and helps you stay on a healthier track, and you'll be less prone to binge eating, which can mentally knock you off course.

While your immediate goal may be to look better in a bathing suit, your long-term vision should focus on being active and healthy in your 70s, 80s, and 90s—not stuck in a wheelchair or laying in a hospital bed, dependant on others for help with your most basic needs.

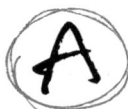

Take Action

Evaluate all the diets you've been on. Are you able to pinpoint a specific diet that worked better for you, both physically and mentally? Was it healthy? If it was, go back and take a peek at it...then work some of the elements into a healthy new lifestyle. Remember, while there are no "bad" foods in a lifestyle change, you still have to make some sacrifices to lose weight. There is no such thing as a free lunch. Pay a little now, reap rewards later.

"Sometimes your body is
smarter than you are."

~ Author Unknown

DAY 15

YOUR HEAD

It's Called Acting:
Fake It

"Life's like a movie, write your own ending.
Keep believing, Keep pretending."
— Jim Henson

Have you ever wondered what it would be like to be someone other than you? Someone without your issues or without your attachment to food or drink? Or someone who truly loves to exercise?

" The beautiful thing about the human mind is its ability to imagine—to fantasize—to transport itself somewhere magical, and for us to become someone we are not. "

Maybe you've never done community theater, but you've probably pretended to be someone else in your life at least a few times. First dates, job interviews, special nights, sports, performances...we've all put on our "game face" at one point or another.

In order to apply this same idea to your weight loss success, you'll need to imagine yourself as the "you" you want to be. The "you" in control of your life, who makes better food choices, exercises consistently, and challenges his/herself. The "you" who is not afraid of change.

Every time you make a food choice, ask yourself: *"What would the 'me I'd like to be' do?"* Each time you want to skip exercise, ask yourself, *"Would the 'me I want to be' do that?"*

I know it sounds corny (and I felt weird at first doing this), but it really does work. You know what to do—envision the "you you would want to be" making all the right choices... choices that help you lose weight, get fitter, and move on with your life.

When the "current you" has a moment of weakness, call on the "me I'd like to be."

The "you that you want to be" is inside you. Trust me. Just coax him or her out, set him free, and become that balanced person you long to be. Adopt the "you's" habits. Live its life. Merge with it. After all—it's still you.

"Fake it 'til you feel it."

It works.

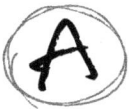 **Take Action**

Make a note (mental or written) of all the qualities the "you you want to be" would have. What would he/she eat? How would he/she cope under stress? What would he/she do if too tired to exercise? Write at least seven positive traits this "perfect you" would have. Each time you encounter a situation where the "current you" is having issues, dig into the "you you want to be's" bag of tricks and try to get yourself over the hump.

THE **DAYS**

DAY 15   Getting to Full

YOUR BODY

A popular diet plan a few years ago encouraged dieters to eat large volumes of foods that fill you up with fewer calories. There's definitely something to that, because when you feel full you're not as likely to continue to eat like you're a starving zombie in a zombie apocalypse. There are foods that naturally make you feel fuller with fewer calories, and then there are foods that pack a lot of calories into a small package, leaving you hungry.

Your mission, should you choose to accept it, is to help yourself feel full. The easiest way to do that?

- Eat your vegetables and salad first, before you touch anything else. They help you feel fuller early on in your meal so you're less likely to eat too much.
- Drink a full glass of water before each meal.
- Try mixing in vegetables and fruits with a high water content, like lettuce, cucumbers, tomatoes, celery, cantaloupe, and oranges.
- Make a low-fat vegetable-filled soup to snack on when you are hungry, or before your main course. Add some beans, too, for additional fiber (and take a little side of the food enzyme alpha galactosidase to prevent gassiness).
- Add vegetables to your main dishes, too, like pastas, pizzas, sandwiches, and egg dishes. The more vegetable-based volume you can create, the better.

- Indulge in whole-grain breads and grains, brown rice, and whole-grain/high-fiber pastas only. Stay away from the "white stuff."
- Eat more soft, or blended, foods like soups, oatmeal, and vegetable/lean protein stews.
- Try a cup of green tea with your meal. It will fill you up, warm your stomach, give you more energy, and possibly boost your metabolism.
- Add lean protein to every meal and snack. Protein keeps you full longer.

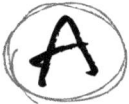

Take Action

Incorporate one of the above bullet items every day, adding a new one day-by-day until you reach the end of the list. You will probably be consistently full more than you've ever been before, and you'll still lose weight. Fill'er up.

THE **DAYS**

DAY
16

"Exercise is a dirty word. Every time
I hear it, I wash my mouth out
with chocolate."

~ Unknown

DAY 16

When the Scale Stops Moving: Hold On

YOUR HEAD

One day, inevitably, the scale stops moving. No matter how hard you work, it seems, or how well you manage your diet, eventually you hit a plateau—and that, my friends, is the ultimate test of your determination.

It's easy to give up. It's easy to wave the white flag and say "*I'll never lose weight*," and go right back to your old habits.

But if you've come this far, don't let a plateau get the best of you. Don't let all those hours spent exercising or all the sugary foods you didn't eat haunt your every waking hour as you contemplate surrender.

Remember this: your body doesn't want you to lose weight. It wants you to hoard fat for the famine that it thinks is coming. It will sabotage you any way it can.

Who will win? You or your body? If you stick with it, you *will* succeed. You might need to just outwait, outsmart, and out-determine your body.

There are also many factors outside of your control that can affect your weight. Your genes, weight loss background, size, and medical history can all work for or against you. The secret sauce that "de-stalls" your body might be to take a moment to review all of these factors, what has worked/

not worked in the past, and make tweaks and adjustments to what you are currently doing.

Before you throw in the towel, remember this: your body wants to win. Keep thinking, keep being creative, and keep going. It doesn't matter whether your weight is temporarily standing still or dropping. You are still progressing.

- No one or diet is perfect
- Expect an occasional setback
- Keep your eye on the ball
- Strive to improve every day
- Don't ever give up

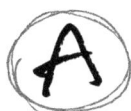

Ⓐ Take Action

Ask yourself:
- Have you adjusted your calorie intake as you've "shrunk" in size? (A smaller body needs fewer calories.)
- Have you fallen into an eating/exercise pattern that has become predictable to your body? (Maybe it's time to shake things up again – see Day 12.)
- Have you changed any medications? (Some medications can really affect your weight.)
- Are you having more "higher calorie days" or eating more of your favorite foods than you should? (Might be time to cut back for a couple of weeks and see what happens.)
- Are you sleeping less than usual or are you more stressed than usual? (Lack of sleep or increased stress can often throw your body out of whack.)

DAY 16 — Quick Workout Ideas to Jumpstart Your Body

YOUR BODY

We're trying to stay on the treadmill of life that keeps going faster and faster. Sometimes, we simply run out of time for longer workouts.

Instead of living in the black-and-white, all-or-nothing world, borrow from what we discussed in previous chapters and fit what you can into your life.

A little bit, done hard, can work miracles on your body.

- Walking on a treadmill for hours on end is great for your overall health, but it's not going to do that much to stoke your fat burning furnace. You need to work focused and targeted. Pick a challenging activity such as cycling, running, swimming or step aerobics to supplement your strength training. Work in hard intervals to get the most results in a shorter amount of time.
- Add plyometric intervals like jump squats, knee tucks, or side jumps to your strength training. Any move that adds a bit of "air" under your feet can be a plyometric.
- Do exercises that use multiple muscles at once: push-ups, squats, lunges, walking lunges, planks, ropes, and pull-ups. (For those of us who can't do pull-ups—myself included—the assisted pull-up machines at many gyms are amazing.) These types of exercises burn more calories, get your heart rate up, and work more of your body faster. You get more for less.

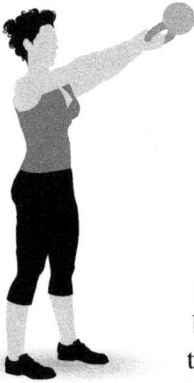

The best of both worlds? Kettlebell training. Kettlebells are incredibly challenging cardiovascularly, and also champions at strengthening your muscles (you'll get a nicely rounded butt and sculpted shoulders). Kettlebell training burns a ton of calories and turns you into a fat-burning machine. Just make sure you receive proper guidance before you start, because while kettlebells are a super way to get in shape, they can also cause injuries if not done correctly.

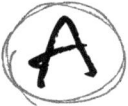

THE **DAYS**

Take Action

When you strength train this week, stop between every two exercises and add deeper squats, lifting your arms up over your head, coming up to your toes as you rise up. Or grab a 5 to 8-pound weighted ball and toss it up in the air as you squat, catching it as you squat down. If you do this consistently between exercises you will start really burning some calories. A happy double-whammy.
(See next page for more exercise illustrations.)

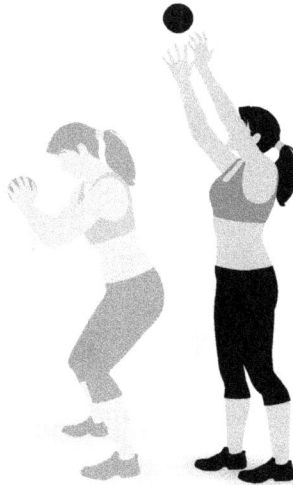

Quick Workouts

Knee Tucks

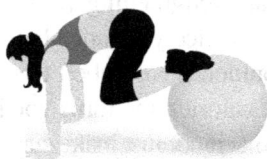

Wall Squat

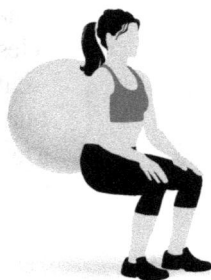

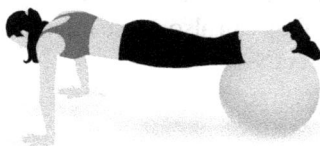

Ball Plank

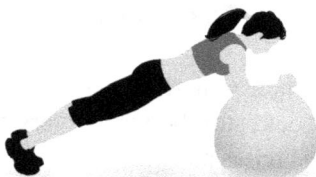

Ball Pushup

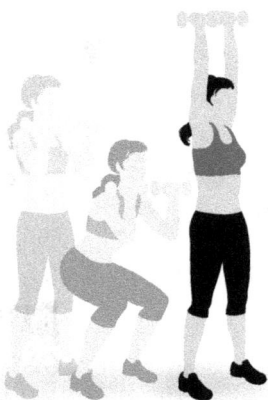

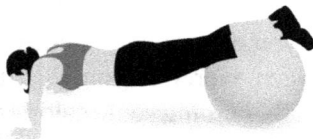

Squat Pressups

DAY
17

"Diets, like clothes, should be
tailored to you."

~Joan Rivers

DAY 17

YOUR HEAD

Saboteurs: OMG Becky

*"It's never your enemies that get you
...it's always your own people."*
~Unknown

How many times have friends or your significant other, knowing you were on a "diet," tried to feed you something you really shouldn't be eating? How many times have you heard, *"Just this once won't hurt,"* or, *"You're obsessed. You look fine. Have another serving."*

As much as friends and family can be your greatest support system during weight loss, they can also be your greatest saboteurs.

Why? Because of the "C Word": change.

As you start taking care of yourself and your weight begins to drop, you would expect the people around you to be happy for you. In some ways they are.

But in other ways they are envious, irritated, or just plain uncomfortable with your progress and may, subconsciously or not, look for ways to sabotage you.

Your friends and family may admire the positive changes you are making, but since they themselves are often not doing anything to improve their own lives you are the most logical target for their guilt. They miss the "fun times" you used to have, don't understand why you want to go to the gym instead of happy hour, or why you choose steamed veggies over their onion rings.

Your new life might be stressing them out because they feel out of control and not capable of making changes in their own lives. Your significant other may be afraid you'll leave them if you look and feel better, and your friends might fear you'll look at them differently or find new friends that share your passion for health. It's all about the potential loss of their status quo—not the gain of your health.

What do you do?

First of all, forgive them. They care about you and don't want to lose what they have—you. They are not being mean, nor are they willfully trying to hurt you. They are trying to keep everything the same as it was and has always been. Change is scary for them, even if it's *you* that's changing.

Stay firm and stick to your guns. If you don't want to eat something, don't eat it. Do not give in to your mother's guilty admonishments, your sister's ridiculing, or your best friend's underhanded remarks.

" You are doing this for you. Period. Do not elaborate. Do not explain. You are in charge your life and what you eat. "

If you have to, stay clear of happy hour with your friends for awhile until you feel strong enough to say *no* consistently.

Or turn down some of those family dinners. Get your blood-work results, and if you have high cholesterol or volatile blood sugar, use those facts to back you up. People can't legitimately frown on medical issues.

In all reality, being fat often boils down to one thing: for whatever your reason, you have a problem controlling your eating and staying motivated to exercise. If you have been able to conquer the beast and come this far, no one has a right to take that control away from you. If you were an alcoholic, they wouldn't tell you, "One drink won't hurt," would they? Because with you and me—one cookie can hurt, at least until we get stronger.

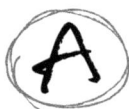

Ⓐ Take Action

Start playing with new friends occasionally. If you work out at a gym, start making acquaintances there who believe in the same healthier lifestyle that you do. I'm not suggesting you ditch your current friends, but rather just expand your friend base. People who are already working out and eating healthy will not try to sabotage you—they see the same big picture as you do. There's nothing wrong with broadening your circle of influence.

Enjoy the Ride — and the Bite

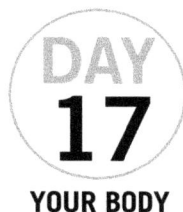

When was the last time you "stopped to smell the food?"

When my children were little I would wolf my food down in 30 seconds before they needed something or a crisis occurred. Now, my children are no longer small and I am still wolfing down my food. Why? It's become a bad habit.

Many people, especially those who are overweight, eat very fast. We find that we don't have much time, we are overly hungry, or we are just afraid that the food will vanish if we don't eat it now.

The problem with this is that by eating too fast you tend to eat too much. It takes anywhere from 10 to 45 minutes from when you begin eating until you start to feel full, and you can do a lot of calorie damage in that time period.

As The Pointer Sisters once sang, "*I want a man with slow hand*." How to find your own slow hand?

- *Enjoy each bite.*
  Take a moment to enjoy the food you are eating. Take smaller bites and really taste your food.
- *Focus on what you are doing.*
  If you're watching television while you are eating, for example, you often don't realize that you've polished off the entire bag of chips until it's too late. In addition

to watching your portion sizes (see Day 3), focus on what you are actually doing: eating.

- *Put the fork down in between.*
  In between every few bites, put the fork down. Grab a sip of water. Or take a break and chat for a few moments. Find a way to slow yourself down until you can start registering some fullness.
- *Try harder-to-eat foods.*
  To slow down naturally, pick foods that require more work, like shelled nuts, soybeans in the pod, and oranges in the peel. It's much easier to eat too many calories by grabbing handfuls of peanuts instead of peanuts in a shell. It's also easier to eat more loose candies than individually wrapped chocolates.
- *Try chopsticks.*
  The ultimate in slowing down? If you are not very skilled with chopsticks they are the perfect utensil to use.

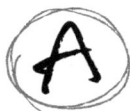

Take Action

At one of your meals today, purposefully drag it out. You might not have a lot of time, but really focus on eating slower, chewing your food well, sipping between bites, and putting your fork down. How long does it take you to start feeling satisfied? Make a mental note of the time. When you are feeling starved in the future, know that this is how long it will take you to feel fuller, and hang on.

DAY
18

"We do not stop exercising because
we grow old – we grow old because
we stop exercising."

~ Dr. Kenneth Cooper

DAY 18
YOUR HEAD

Save Yourself with Some Planning

"Failing to plan is planning to fail"
~ Alan Lakein

If you've ever found yourself desperately headed for a drive-through (for a double something with extra fries and a large shake on the side) because you desperately needed to eat or you'd rip someone's face off, this is the chapter for you: saving yourself through a bit of planning.

In my personal life, I am not a big planner overall. I like to fly by the seat of my pants and take things as they come. However, one thing I have learned through my whole weight-loss journey is that you have to plan in order to be successful.

If you didn't eat enough for breakfast, or skipped lunch completely, you are familiar with the hunger and fatigue demon that rears its head right around 3 p.m. That's when anything from stale donuts to a bag of chips are all fair game....and that will challenge your efforts to lose weight.

The idea? Plan ahead and come up with ideas and strategies that set you up for success—not failure.

1. Shop or go on errands on a fairly full belly. Even if it's 10 a.m. and you think you'll be back in time for lunch, Murphy's law says you might not make it. Grab a de-

cent snack (preferably protein) before you go to make sure you're not facing the world famished.

2. Have healthy, little snacks on hand that you can bring with you on errands, to school, or to work. Nuts, whole-grain crackers with peanut butter, or carrots all do the trick to take the edge off your hunger. Even a protein bar will do in a pinch (though many are heavy on sugar—read labels). Something semi-healthy in your belly beats onion rings any day.

3. Keep snacks ready to go at home, too. Low-fat string cheese, cottage cheese, fresh veggies, a hardboiled egg, or a bit of shredded chicken or turkey slices are really good snacking options. (See more snack ideas Day 20: Healthy Snacks.)

4. Don't eat food/snack items directly from their original container. How many times have you intended to eat only a few chips and then realized only later that half the bag is gone? Put a reasonable portion in a bowl, then put the bag away.

5. Eat a snack before going to a restaurant. I know it sounds counterintuitive, but having a light salad, a lean protein, or some raw veggies can save you from filling up on chips or bread when eating out.

6. Before attending any party or gathering, do the same as #5, above.

Planning...
it just takes
a moment

THE **DAYS**

By planning just a bit ahead, you'll give yourself that extra bit of help to make sure that this time you succeed.

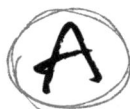

(A) Take Action

Make sure this week that you have healthy snacks planned and available. Eat before you go out, snack wisely at work, and don't let yourself get too hungry. Pay attention to how it feels when snacking becomes a good thing. You might very well stop craving the "nutrition-light" variety.

Give Yourself a Challenge

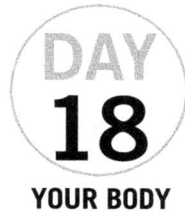

"Help, I'm alive..."
     ~Metric

There are times a day or so after a really hard workout, that I really do feel like saying, *"Help, I'm alive!"* because my muscles are so sore that I cannot sit easily.

That level of muscle soreness (DOMS—or delayed onset muscle soreness) is rare if you've been working out for awhile, but when you first start an exercise program or change up your workout it's a familiar feeling. Good pain, as we often say in the workout world.

> Help prevent muscle soreness by immersing yourself in a cold bath or pool right after exercising.

How can pain be good? For one simple reason: you know your muscles have been worked. Who cares about the science behind it or why we feel sore? Who cares if it really means anything? The true value of DOMS is how it makes us feel emotionally: we have done something for us, our bodies, and our minds. This one day our muscles are screaming with every movement; it is a day that we have broken free of past patterns, defied the odds, and moved our bodies in a way they aren't used to.

When you work out, make sure you really challenge yourself. Maybe not to the extreme of constantly feeling DOMS, but so that you truly feel you've done something. If you've ever watched those people at the gym whose bodies never change, year after year, you might notice a pattern: they are working at half effort, reading a magazine or just chatting their way through their workouts or classes. If you have that kind of time to kill, then more power to you. But if, like the rest of us, your time is very tight, you want to make it count. You're exercising for a reason: to lose weight, get in shape, and strengthen your heart, lungs, and body—not your mouth.

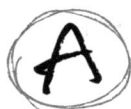

Ⓐ Take Action

At your next workout (even if it's at home or on a walk), really focus on the work you are doing. Feel your muscles contract and extend. When you've reached what you think is your max repetitions, do two more. Work extra hard your last 10 minutes of cardio. You will be surprised how much farther you can go when you push one step at a time.

DAY
19

"Feeding is a very important ritual
for me. I don't trust people who
don't like to eat."

~Gina Gershon

DAY 19
Staying on Track: Move Along

YOUR HEAD

"And even when your hope is gone, move along, move along just to make it through."
All American Rejects

Invariably there will come a time when you just get tired of eating healthy and exercising.

Day after day of commitment, saying "yes" to good choices and "no" to poor choices, might wear you down. Maybe you're just in the mood for a really good cry—or a really long binge.

" Whatever it is, just know this is normal. "

You are not a failure for getting tired of always being on your toes and thinking ahead, or for always getting up early to fit in your exercise. As human beings, every now and then we want to have fun and indulge our "id" (the childlike part of us that "wants it now" and craves pleasure and entertainment).

Being truly successful with weight loss involves a whole lifestyle change, and this isn't always easy. You have to change your complete relationship to food, thought patterns, eating, exercise, sleeping, etc. You have to learn how to solve problems without overeating, to not feed your hungry heart, and to exercise when it's easier to just stay in bed. You have to constantly be on the lookout for weight loss traps.

When you feel like you've reached a wall, give yourself a little something. Take a week off from exercise (gasp!) or do something different. Add in one day when you just eat whatever comes along, but *not* purposefully binging (just relax your standards for that day). Take a few days and don't obsess about how much you exercised or how many glasses of water you drank. Just let things flow naturally.

Your overall goal is to learn to give your body what it needs to be healthy — not to live by numbers and obsessions. Constantly thinking about food choices, learning better habits, and educating yourself about portion sizes are all a necessary part of learning your new lifestyle but once they are ingrained in you, then you should not have to think about things quite so hard.

Discover a healthier way of living...and then let it all come organically from there. That is the way you keep yourself on track. If you start to slip too far, just tighten things up until you find yourself where you need to be.

- Don't fight with food
- Don't fight with your body
- There are no "bad" foods — only too much of any one thing
- Learn balance and get rid of obsessions

Life is indeed too short to fret.

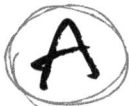

A) Take Action

Take a moment and stop fretting. Borrow a holistic approach and feel "at one" with your body...and just let it be.

DAY 19 Sleep Your Way Thin

YOUR BODY

We're told we need to sleep eight hours each night, and while that's true for many people, it's not true for everyone.

What is true for most people is that sleeping too little really may cause you to gain weight, or slow down your weight loss.

Not getting enough sleep is both emotionally and chemically crippling to your desire to lose weight. When you're really tired and your tank is empty, it's a natural impulse to make yourself feel better by downing a caffeinated, sugar-filled drink or a bag of chips and a donut. The sugar and caffeine rush gets you going again—until you crash. When you're running on lack of sleep and lots of sugar, you also have no energy to exercise. So, the pounds start to come on.

Deep inside your body, though, your lack of sleep is sabotaging you in other ways. Your metabolism stops working as efficiently, and your hormones go awry. Leptin, the friendly hormone, is the one that tells you when you are full. When you don't sleep enough, your Leptin levels drop so you want to eat more. Ghrelin, on the other hand, tells you when you are hungry. Ghrelin levels rise when you aren't getting enough sleep, so your body tells you "eat, eat."

A simple equation tells us that higher levels of "eat" hormone coupled with lower levels of "don't eat" hormone, with an added splash of lowered metabolism, can equal disaster to your waistline. However, don't use this as an excuse not to try. I was able to lose most of my weight while still not sleeping enough. You just have to be smart about it. Sleep when you can. Don't reach for unhealthy snacks. Work out more. Nothing revitalizes a tired body better than exercise.

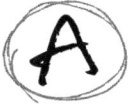

Take Action

The sleep you get before midnight is the most valuable, so attempt to go to bed just a little earlier this week. Even 30 minutes will make a difference. If you're like me and tend to pull late nights working, try going to bed earlier and getting up earlier to work out. It's no fun sliding out of bed at 5 a.m. when it's pitch black outside, but if you went to bed an hour earlier than usual, it might just help you lose weight.

THE **DAYS**

DAY
20

"He who has health, has hope. And he who has hope, has everything."

~Proverb

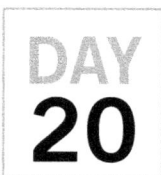

DAY 20
YOUR HEAD

So Much More: Meant to Live

"We were meant to live for so much more, have we lost ourselves?"
~Switchfoot

I remember snapping at a concerned friend a few years ago. It was during my divorce and I hadn't talked to her for awhile. We went out to lunch and she asked me how things were going with the divorce. Since I felt like this was all I had been talking about with anyone for months I hissed, "I am *more* than my divorce."

The moral of that story is that you are *more* than your weight. Whether fat, thin, or in between, you have much more to offer the world than thinking or talking about weight. There are people to feed, lives to change, customers to make happy, children to raise, art to paint, poetry to write, and songs to dance to. But sometimes, when you are struggling with your weight, you become it. You, in fact, are so very much more.

Being successful with weight loss doesn't only affect your health and appearance—it also affects your mind. The more weight you lose, and the fitter you get, the stronger your mind becomes, and that's when true change takes place.

It's not too far-fetched to say that losing weight and getting in shape changes lives, but it changes them in ways that aren't so visible. Once you become free of your obsession with food, a whole new world opens up to you. Once you log hours running, cycling, or in the gym—sometimes truly bored out of your mind but still forging ahead—you learn that nothing is impossible.

When you have reached your fitness and weight goals and have stayed on track for awhile, it's an opportunity to break the focus away from you and your body, and start looking at ways you can help others. What advice can you impart? What stories can you share? Whose life can you make easier?

This is why I became a trainer and group exercise instructor (and returned to my writing roots). Once I stopped focusing on my weight—once I broke out of the negative prison I found myself in—I saw clearly that my experience could help others break free as well. Through trial, error, and blood, sweat, and tears I was able to accomplish something major. I wanted to share that success with others and watch them succeed too. Teach, motivate, and watch them fly.

I was meant to live for so much more than eating ice cream at 1 a.m.

You are, too.

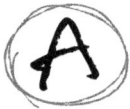 **Take Action**

Think about what you can do to make the lives around you better.

DAY 20
Healthy, Fun Snacking

YOUR BODY

Snacking will save you.

I am not talking about the "*100 calorie snacking packs*" out there (though if it's between that and a side of fries, the snack pack would win).

I exercise a lot so I am often hungry. Maybe I am also hungry because I went without structured meals for much of my early life. I don't know. All I know is that I don't like to feel too hungry.

Snacking has many benefits when it comes to weight loss. It helps keep you from overeating later, keeps your energy up, and helps your brain function.

Snacks have to be healthy, though. You want to stay away from as many refined carbohydrates (junkie-type foods) and sugars as possible, because sugar makes you crave more sugar. If you are craving something sweet, you do have options and some leeway. Just try to balance out anything "carb-y" or sugary with a protein.

Snacking = Binge preventer

Snack Suggestions

Healthy Snacks
- Low-fat string cheese
- Fat-free cottage cheese
- Plain Greek yogurt (add some berries for sweetness)
- Nuts (in moderation)
- Olives (in moderation)
- Low-fat turkey slices or shredded chicken
- Hardboiled Eggs
- Raw vegetables (anything and everything)
- Hummus
- Protein smoothie (but watch the sugars)

Curb-a-Craving Snack
- Apple slices with peanut butter
- Trail mix (but be cautious of how much)
- Strawberries with a drizzle of chocolate and a side dipping of plain yogurt
- Berries (with a dash of low-fat whipped cream)
- Low-fat graham crackers with low-fat cream cheese
- Dark chocolate square with peanut butter

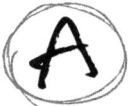

Take Action

Stock your pantry and fridge with more from the first list, and just a few from the second. Try to reach for the Healthy Snacks items when at all possible. If a craving strikes and you are about to dive into the jelly beans, go for items on the *Curb-a-Craving Snack list* instead to quell the sugar monster.

DAY
21

"An hour of basketball feels like 15 minutes. An hour on a treadmill feels like a weekend in traffic school."

~ David Walters

DAY 21

Tips &Tricks: All the Small Things

YOUR HEAD

"If I'd observed all the rules, I'd never have got anywhere."
~Marilyn Monroe

The Golden Rules cheat sheet. Here are the most important things you need to remember...in one place.

- **Brush your teeth** (or use a strong mouthwash) after every meal. It gets the taste of food out of your mouth so you don't crave more, and you won't want to "dirty" your clean mouth again.

- **Start out with smaller goals** and don't go all "Kill Bill" on yourself. When you sacrifice too much too fast you burn out and lose the desire to go on. If you overdo exercise, your constantly sore muscles will try to knock you off your path. Start at about 50% of where you normally would. It took a long time to gain the weight— it's going to take awhile to get rid of it. Right now, your fat and you are pretty good buddies. Part slowly.

- **Wear tighter clothes.** Buy at least one pair of pants that are snug at the waist and wear them frequently. The snugness will remind you why you are doing all this, and will also show you quickly when you start to see results. Sweatpants, my friend, have been many a person's downfall.

- **Set small goals** and celebrate each one that you reach (with something other than food). Think of your life as scales of justice, with failures on one side and successes on the other. For many of us, we have failed so many times at weight loss that our "failure side" is far outweighing the "success side." Building in small successes will slowly start to even out those scales, and hopefully one day your "success side" will outweigh the "failure side" (pun intended).

- **Don't think in black or white**. Even if you've eaten half a tray of cupcakes you haven't "blown it." Throw the box away (far away), go brush your teeth, maybe exercise, and, most importantly, don't beat yourself up. Just forget it ever happened. Don't let one wrong move throw you off course. You're bigger than that.

- **You always have a choice**—use it positively. You have the choice to say "no" to food and "yes" to exercise. Remember, every time someone "drives" you to eat (yes, we've all thought that way) the other person wins. Not you. You are the one sitting there in misery, with a hurting stomach, gas, and heartburn. The other person? They're not suffering....not one bit. Stop hurting yourself.

- **Take yourself and your health seriously**. You only have one life and one chance. Make it count.

THE **DAYS**

131

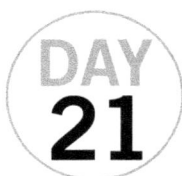

DAY 21 — Fix Your Broken Metabolism

YOUR BODY

If years of dieting and lack of strength training have taken their toll on your body, your metabolism may be feeling wrecked.

Unless there's a medical issue (or you are taking certain types of medication), you can give your metabolism a quick kick in the rear. When your weight loss has hit a plateau, it's time for change.

- **Food**
  Start eating more for a couple of weeks. Then slowly begin to eat less for a week. See where you are. If you are not losing weight, cut your calories a bit more, or increase your exercise. Work to find a balance of what works, then start calorie cycling.
- **Eat more often and more high protein foods**
  Proteins take more energy to digest, and also help you feel full longer. And every time you eat, you stimulate your metabolism a little.
- **Exercise**
  Try to exercise more overall. Exercise not only burns calories instantly but also gives you an "afterburn" that keeps you burning calories long after you're done.
- **Add more intervals** to your aerobic workouts. The recovery period after your interval training helps you burn more calories.

- **Start with some heavy strength training** to put on muscle. When you lift heavier weights, your body uses more energy to repair the (normal) microscopic tears to the muscle. Muscle also needs more calories to survive than fat does, so you burn more calories throughout the day.
- **Fidget or move**
  People who physically move a lot or fidget burn about 300 additional calories per day. So if you pace while talking on the phone, tap your feet, gesture, fidget, park farther away, take stairs instead of the elevator, get up from your desk every 30 minutes, or just simply walk from point A to point B, you will increase the calories you use almost effortlessly.
- **Keep cool**
  Being a bit cool forces your body to use more energy just to keep warm. Your appetite also seems to be less when you're not as comfortable.

In the beginning, when you increase your food and lift heavier weights, your weight might actually go up. Don't fret. This is temporary and can help re-set your body and metabolism. In a couple of weeks you should start seeing your weight drop again. Don't give up and don't starve yourself—starving is your metabolism's worst enemy.

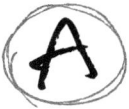

Take Action

Start fidgeting and moving. This week, get up from your desk (or sofa) every 30 minutes and spend 2 minutes moving fairly briskly. If you have steps, walk up and down them a few times. Just move, all the time.

Resources

Help is On The Way

Useful links
Articles
Inspiration
Day-by-day journal

FOOD GUIDE

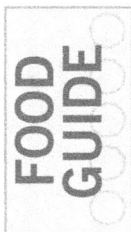

An Insider's Guide to Food
(a supplement to Day 1 – Your Body)

What's in a name? Plenty! And it can be plenty confusing, too. Below is a real life breakdown of what the main food components are, why you need them and where to find them.

(Need help with calculations? Let's put on our math hats. Take a 2,000-calorie diet, for example. If you want to eat 25% protein per day, use the 2,000 and multiply by .25 — just add a decimal before the percentage — which will give you 500 calories from protein. Divide 500 calories by 4 (there are 4 calories per gram of protein), and your "magic" daily protein number would be 125 grams if you choose 25%.)

Don't get discouraged if you don't understand all of this. There are many (often free) online calculators that can calculate for you. *See next page for links and help.*

- **Carbohydrates (4 calories per gram):**
  WHAT THEY DO: Carbohydrates are broken down into sugars (glucose) for immediate energy needs, with extras stored as glycogen for longer-term energy and brain function.
  WHERE THEY ARE FOUND: Fruits, vegetables, legumes (beans, lentils, and peanuts), and whole grains (plus of course cakes, cookies, candy, etc.).
  HOW MUCH TO EAT: 45–65% of your daily calories (though many weight loss professionals recommend in the 50% or less range).

- **Proteins (4 calories per gram):**
  WHAT THEY DO: Proteins help give you energy, rebuild
  your body, and make you feel fuller longer.
  WHERE THEY ARE FOUND: Lean meats and poultry,
  seafood, low-fat dairy products (cottage cheese, yogurt,
  milk, and cheeses), eggs, beans, lentils, quinoa, and nuts
  HOW MUCH TO EAT: 10–35% from protein (though
  many weight loss professionals recommend staying in
  the 20–25% range.)

- **Fiber:**
  WHAT IT DOES: Fiber reduces the risk of developing
  coronary heart disease, stroke, high blood pressure,
  diabetes, obesity, and some gastrointestinal diseases
  WHERE IT IS FOUND: Whole-grain products, fruits,
  vegetables, beans, peas, nuts and seeds
  HOW MUCH TO EAT: 22–28 grams per day for women,
  28–34 grams for males

- **Fats (9 calories per gram):**
  WHAT THEY DO: "Healthy" dietary fat provides energy
  and is a building block for your cell membranes. Fats
  digest slower so they keep you full longer. Some vita-
  mins are fat-soluble only (like A, D, E, and K), which
  means they dissolve in fat and can be stored in your body.
  WHERE THEY ARE FOUND: Unsaturated fats, such as
  lean poultry, fish, and olive-, nut-, and canola oils
  HOW MUCH TO EAT: 20–35% from fat (though many
  weight loss and health care professionals recommend
  under 30%)

RESOURCES

LINKS

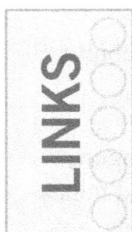

Calculators, Online Nutrition Information, Weight Loss Programs & Groups

NUTRITION AND CALORIE CALCULATORS
www.HealthCalculators.org
www.mayoclinic.com/health/calorie-calculator/NU00598
www.Nutrition.gov
www.Nutrition.org
www.CDC.gov/HealthyWeight/
www.EatRight.org/Public/

ONLINE DIET PROGRAMS AND RESOURCES
Not only do these sites offer provide tons of resources, calculators, menu plans, and educational articles, but some of them feature bona fide healthy, balanced diets.

www.mayoclinic.com/health/weight-loss/MY00432
www.SparkPeople.com
www.WeightWatchers.com
www.WebMD.com/diet
www.EDiets.com
www.DietWatch.com
www.SouthBeachDiet.com
www.DukeDiet.com

WEIGHT LOSS SUPPORT AND COMMUNITY
Support groups and discussion forums to answer your
questions and share experiences.
www.fitnessrepublic.com
www.SparkPeople.com
www.3FatChicks.com
www.Diet.com

COOKING AND RECIPES FOR WEIGHT LOSS
www.CookingLight.com/
www.EatingWell.com
www.Hungry-Girl.com
www.MyRecipes.com/healthy-recipes
www.3FatChicks.com/diet-recipes

www.ThisMamaCooks.com

EXERCISE TOOLS & RESOURCES
www.ACEFitness.org/getfit
www.FitnessMagazine.com
www.Shape.com
www.WomensHealthMag.com
www.MensHealth.com
www.OxygenMag.com
www.iVillage.com/diet-fitness

TRAINER/INSTRUCTOR LOCATORS
www.FitnessConnect.com (certified trainer locator)
www.DragonDoor.com (RKC kettlebell instructors locator)

(For "live" links that you can click through to, visit my
blog at www.realworldweightloss.com/21daysbook.)

RESOURCES

FITNESS

Your Heart Rate: Ma'am, Do you Know How Fast You Were Going?

Exercising aerobically without a heart rate monitor is much like driving a car without a speedometer. Doesn't make much sense, now does it?

Monitoring your heart rate measures your exercise intensity—the harder the work, the higher the heart rate (though other factors, such as the shape you are in and medications like beta blockers do come into play).

Many people use the simple "rate of perceived exertion" (or RPE) to measure exercise intensity. RPE is just your own opinion of how hard an activity feels to *you* while you're actually doing it. The downside to RPE is that it's not entirely accurate. There are other factors that affect your RPE versus how hard you are actually working, like how much sleep you've gotten, how much you've worked out that week, and if you're a woman, where in your menstrual cycle you are.

Measuring your actual heart rate (rather using than RPE) helps you vary the intensity of your exercise. (Remember the Shock! Method?) Some days you want to exercise at a steady rate, building your stamina and burning more fat as your energy source. Other days you want to do harder intervals, increasing your power and heart output, while burning more calories.

(Side note: though there's debate about fat-burning zones versus interval training, aerobic zones from 70–85% of your maximum heart rate do use more fat as primary fuel to keep you going. Intervals, on the other hand—working in the 65%-92% range—use more of your muscles' sugars. However, intervals burn more calories overall than steady-state aerobic training, so in all reality—in terms of weight loss—they are the same. You need both for variety and to train and shock your body).

Ready to put your heart rate to the test? Buy an inexpensive heart rate monitor. (Get the least expensive base model that does nothing but measure your heart rate. It doesn't tell you how many calories you've burned, which is not accurate, anyway, and won't cook your dinner. It simply tells you how hard you are working.)

Go to the links below and calculate your maximum and working zone heart rates (65%, 75%, 85%, and 92%). For more accuracy, take a look at the "Karvonen method" of calculating your individual training zones. General heart rate recommendations are not that accurate, and Karvonen gives you a better number tailored to you.

To know your body is to know your heart rate.

Heart rate calculators:
www.active.com/fitness/calculators/heartrate.htm
walking.about.com/cs/calories/l/blcalcheartrate.htm

Karvonen method of calculating heart rate (preferred):
www.sparkpeople.com/resource/calculator_target.asp
www.fitwatch.com/qkcalc/thr.html

RESOURCES

FITNESS

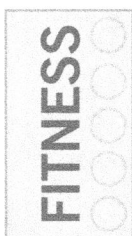

Strength Training Tips: The Buff Zone

- **Lift a heavy enough weight** so that you can do a minimum of 8 repetitions and a maximum of 18 repetitions. If you can perform more than 18 repetitions without struggling, increase the weight (unless you are doing a high repetition/lower weight session to shake things up.).

- **Superset your exercises.** For example, the back works in conjunction with the biceps, so work the back, then the biceps, the chest and the triceps, and so on.

" In order to improve and get more toned, you have keep increasing the weight or the challenge. "

- **Split your workouts if you are short on time.** Work your upper body one day, your buns, legs and abdominals another. 15-20 minutes should more than cover an upper body or a lower body/abdominal routine. Just work hard.

- **Don't stop at a certain number.** If you tell yourself you are doing 15 repetitions of an exercise and your muscle is not extremely tired when you get to 15, keep going! Make a mental note of how many reps you actully do, and then adjust your weight up for next time.

- **Pay attention to your speed and form.** Don't go too fast. A good speed is two counts on the concentric part (shortening of the muscle) with four counts on the eccentric (lengthening of the muscle).

> *What does this mean?* With a bicep curl, for example, take two counts to lift the weight up (concentric) and four counts to lower it (eccentric). The effort is faster, the return is slower. You can vary your training with static holds at the bottom, middle, or top of the exercise, or change up your speed. Some workouts use super slow reps (for example, five counts on the shortening—concentric—and seven counts on the lengthening—eccentric). Or 2-2. Or 1-1. Or you can "explode up," and slowly lower back down again. Vary, vary, vary. That's the ticket to success.

- **Don't rest in between exercises.** Alternate between two movements, for example, so you constantly keep moving and working your muscles.

- **Add a stability challenge**. Work on a BOSU® (half ball), stand on one leg, sit on a stability ball, lift a kettlebell, or be barefoot, use a foam pad, a pillow, or disks (paper plates, furniture movers) that glide.

Muscles don't grow (or "tone up") without proper rest. Let 48 hours pass between strength-training sessions for the same body parts. Allow time for your muscles to regenerate. All work and no rest=no change and a waste of time.

RESOURCES

BRAIN FOOD

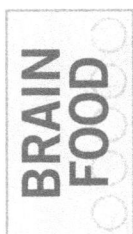

How Much Exercise is Enough to Lose Weight?

The amount of exercise you need a day is a difficult question to answer.

Celebrities often claim to exercise two hours a day. On TV, weight loss shows feature people exercising more than four hours each day. Health advocates say 30 minutes of daily activity is enough to keep you healthy.

So...how much exercise do you really need? With 66% of the U.S. adult population either overweight or obese, weight management has become very important. It seems the more we obsess about weight, the fatter we become. Where "thin is in," we are neither...thin nor healthy.

The American College of Sports Medicine (ACSM), an association of sports medicine, exercise science, and health and fitness professionals, recommends the following amounts of exercise for preventing weight gain and accelerating weight loss.

PREVENTING WEIGHT GAIN

It's easier to keep your weight down than to try to lose what you've already gained. 150 minutes per week of moderate intensity exercise, i.e. walking, is enough to do just that. *Roughly translated, 150 minutes is about 30 minutes a day, five days a week.*

Think that's too much? How much time do you spend watching TV? Surfing the web? Talking on the phone? Sitting at a coffee shop? It's probably more than 30 minutes each day.

" Studies have shown that breaking your exercise session up, for example into three 10-minute bouts, is just as effective as one longer session. "

So walk during your morning break, take the stairs, or walk the kids home from school. Take 10 minutes out for you.

WEIGHT LOSS

More than 150 minutes per week of moderate intensity physical activity is recommended for modest weight loss benefits. However, more than 250 minutes per week provides larger amounts of weight loss.

How much per day is 250 minutes per week? That's about 50 minutes each day, five days a week. Still not that bad. A 20 minute walk in the early morning, 10 minute walk during a break, 20 minute walk after dinner. Or a 1-hour group exercise class four days a week, plus one short walk.

Significant weight loss is worth that minor investment, isn't it?

THE SHORTCUTS

These are ACSM's recommendations for "moderate-intensity physical activity," but as many experts will tell you, there are ways to exercise less and still reap weight loss and health benefits. You have to work smarter, harder, constantly change things up and give it your best...all the time.

RESOURCES

- **Exercise at a higher intensity** to burn more calories overall. Perform intervals while walking, running, or cycling. (Work very hard for 20 seconds, then recover for at least three times that amount, work very hard again, then recover.)

- **Do multiple-muscle or large muscle exercises** (squats, lunges, side steps with bicep curl, full pushups, ball roll-outs), kettlebell training, bootcamps, or circuit training.

- **Strength train.** Like most fitness professionals and organizations, ACSM also recommends strength training as part of a health and fitness regimen in order to increase muscle mass and further reduce health risks.

My general rule of thumb? If you can read a magazine or book while exercising, it's too easy. Focus on the work, and exercise harder, for a shorter time period. Make every minute count. Walk and chat with your friends, sure, as part of your "30-minutes a day" general rule. But work with intensity for weight loss.

"Some people dream of success... while others wake up and work hard at it." ~Author Unknown

Precisely.

Overeating When You Know Better

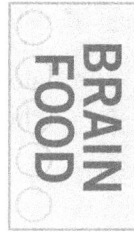

BRAIN FOOD

If you're reading this, you know what I am talking about.

Overeating. Binging. Eating too much, too fast. You know it's bad for you. You know it's unhealthy. You know it will often lead to more and more "bad" days, until once again you can't button your pants. After your eating spree you will wake up feeling bloated, fat, puffy, and sick. It is the overeaters' version of a hangover (the "foodover?"), at which time you ask yourself, *"What was the point of that?"*

The actual process of losing weight is really pretty simple. What's not simple is overcoming the mental obstacles that prevent you from weight loss.

Magazines are full of wonderful and useful tips to help you reduce body fat. Exercise programs with promises of flat abs in mere minutes abound. With health clubs on every corner, we should be a thin and fit nation.

What no one really talks about, though, is the main reason so many of us fail with our weight loss efforts: our minds won't let us.

- Do you often work all day, cook for your family, finish chores, shop, help kids with homework, and watch after-school sporting events—all on five hours of sleep?

- Do you constantly help others, and "go go go" until there's nothing left for you, finally finding yourself alone and exhausted at midnight with your hand in the chip bag?

Are you a bad person for overeating? No.

Are you weak? No.

Let's face it. You are tired. Sometimes the only way you have to relieve pressure is to eat (when only the "bad" foods will do, of course).

So how do you change your habits and get yourself on the weight loss track?

- Know that there are other people out there that feel just like you.

- Know that beating yourself up for being "weak once more" won't help.

- Try to take the power out of food by not thinking about it as much, not obsessing, and not worrying about everything you put in your mouth. (Sounds contradictory to what you have learned in the past, I know. Count calories, count fat, count carbs.)

For now, the above should be all you focus on. Next time you look at the box of donuts, remind yourself that it's just food and that it shouldn't have that kind of power over you. It's not about the donuts. It's about the person who upset you, or the extra work, or the fatigue, or the hopelessness. But sometimes you can't change your immediate situation, so getting annoyed at the box of donuts trying to control you might just help.

Try to overcome the "binge demon" that lurks in your head. If you can stave him off even for an hour or a meal or a day, you have won. For that one moment you have taken your life back. If you fall off the food wagon again, so be it. But cherish that one victory.

Push the food demon around—don't let him push you.

BRAIN FOOD

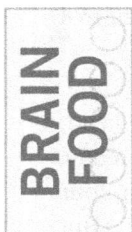

I Love My Thighs: An Essay

Yes, that's correct. You actually heard a woman say that she loves her thighs.

My thighs are not particularly attractive: they are neither long nor thin nor tan. In fact, they are kind of short, bulky, and pale. So why do I love them?

Through literally thick and thin, my legs have done their job. They have climbed to the top of the Acropolis in Greece; splashed in the fjords of Norway; walked on the beaches of Thailand. They have taken me 100 miles by bicycle from Irvine to San Diego, California, run a 5k in Temecula, California, and ridden up the side of a mountain.

These very same legs have rocked babies to sleep, walked children to school, and held kids up in the air in a game of "airplane." As a personal trainer, they have shown clients how good it feels to move, and as a Spinning instructor they have led full classes on endorphin-elevating adventures.

My thighs have seen a lot. They have been very overweight, where at times they would blister on the insides from rubbing together. They have been very thin, where light could actually be seen between them. Now they are in the middle. Neither thin nor fat, but rather sturdy and muscular.

I never feel as great as when I'm wearing bike shorts, mounting a bicycle, feet secured in familiar clipless pedals, thighs ready for action. I'm sure I don't actually look as fabulous as I feel in those bike shorts, but I don't really care—I am strong, capable, and very happy.

Sometimes I wish I had long, lean legs—the kind that turn men's heads. But then I remember that turning men's heads does not make me feel empowered, that wearing a miniskirt well does not release endorphins, and that no amount of tanning will get me up the side of a mountain on a bicycle.

" My thighs have given me freedom. They have taken me interesting places and more adventures lie ahead. There are many foreign beaches to comb and ancient ruins to scale. "

So even if I cannot turn men's heads by the length and beauty of my legs, maybe I can turn their heads by leg pressing their trucks. After all, that would be memorable. *And creating memories are what my legs do.*

Take the Long Way Home

13 Days in the Life of a Diet

From spinach to nacho cravings:.
What it's really like to try to lose
weight. A day-by day journey into
dieting—laughing, crying and
resisting cookies

Dieter's Journal

1

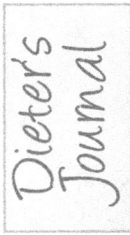

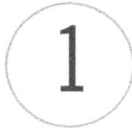

DAY 1: THE STRUGGLE

Six years ago I weighed 116 pounds. A respectable weight for a woman 5' tall. Two years before that I weighed 198 pounds; *not* a respectable weight for a woman my height. Now I weigh 130 pounds and am determined to lose the pounds to get back to my "fighting weight."

I used to rock the free world. Six years ago I was my absolute strongest. I climbed mountains on my bicycle, rode 100 miles in a "century ride," smashed every barrier I knew to prove to myself that I was no longer a big, fat failure. I was a killer Spinning instructor and a rockin' personal trainer. I truly was at the top of my physical game.

What happened to make me lose momentum? I got divorced. Divorce is hard on everyone. Confusion, sadness, poverty... friends and family lost. No need to go into detail—if you have been there you know what it feels like—but over the next few years I let my passion slide...just a little. Then I let my rules relax...just a little. Had some candy here, some chocolate there, some chips over here, brownie batter over there. A little more. Then a little more. A loaf of hot French bread from the store? Break off a huge chunk, slap some cheese on it, and let it take away the stress...for a moment.

THAT OH-SO-MAGICAL MOMENT

The magic moment is the one special time where you do for you and you alone. The moment where you feel special, safe, and taken care of. It doesn't matter if it's a fake moment. In the turmoil that surrounds you it is *your* moment, and no one—no one—can take that away from you. You control the only thing you can: what and how much you eat. So you binge. Aaaah. The moment.

The moment, unfortunately, lasts such a short time. Then you "wake up" to reality and realize that not only did you eat anything and everything you should not have (the carrots are still left untouched in their bag), but you feel terrible. Bloated. And—gasp!—fat again. But you are so tired, so stressed, so overwhelmed with keeping your little household afloat and your career moving forward that you indulge just a bit...and a bit more...and a bit more. Until none of your size 4 pants fit. And your size 6 pants give you muffin top. You wonder. And then you cry.

You try and try again to get "back on the wagon." How can this be so hard? You've already lost 80 pounds. You still teach Spinning and you still train clients. But...you also indulge in far too many "comfort" foods. You are much happier inside being free of your marriage, but the struggle of keeping a roof over your head lets that little voice take over. The voice that says, "*Just a little bit won't hurt. Just a little cookie dough will make you feel sooo good. You deserve it.*" And so you give in.

THE TURNING POINT

Long hours of working at a desk (you are also a freelance writer and a marketing pro), combined with severe lack of sleep and overall exhaustion, land you in urgent care. The doctor finally tells you that you need to sleep (oops, it's 11:45 p.m. again), and slow down. Slowing down is not an option at this point, and you can entertain the sleep thing, but in all reality—you need to start eating healthier again. Take charge of your health, take charge of your life... like you did once before.

So there you are. With your muffin top. Ready to kick some a**. Because you are sick of being tired. And plumpish.

TODAY'S STATS

- 7 hour of sleep. Yay.
- 20 minutes of abdominals/butt work (in my PJs) at home. That's all I could fit in. Had to go easy on the legs because of Spinning class later.

In the evening, taught a 1-hour very hard Spinning class (not in my PJs).

Onward and forward.

Until tomorrow.

2

Dieter's Journal

DAY 2: CHOCOLATE

If you read yesterday's post you would have noted that I was full of vim and vigor and ready to lose weight. Today...today I am tired. And wanting this bag full of loose chocolates sitting in my drawer.

I stayed up too late again last night and am feeling it today. When we are tired, we often turn to sugar to "perk us up." Yes, we know it's a temporary perk but everything in life is temporary, is it not? And though it won't solve anything in the long run, in the short run that sugar rush feels just so fabulous.

Shall I eat those chocolates? No, I shall not. I might have, if I had not started this little public blogging experiment. I'd feel a bit like a cheater if I wrote all these motivating things, and then secretly scarfed down the bag of chocolates.

THE 3:30 DEATHTRAP

I will say that the doctor was right. I need more sleep. I should not have stayed up working until 12:30 a.m., and arisen early this morning. But I did and now, at 3:30 p.m. I am suffering. I am back at my desk trying to work and my eyes are slipping closed. I will try an apple and some green tea, as though that would take the place of coffee and chocolate.

JOURNAL

I know very well that if I can hang with it for the next hour my sleepiness and sugar cravings will go away. I will try hard. I am determined. My pants are too tight. But right now I am safely dressed in sweatpants—another reason I regained some of that weight. Sweatpants are the devil and you can't feel your weight gain in them.

HANGIN' WITH IT

It seems that the 82 pounds I lost were easy compared to this. Was I that much younger? Was I that much stronger? Or was I that much closer to the realization that I won't live forever?

Women are motivated by emotional trauma and men by medical concerns. It's been years since my father died and I think that "reality-blow" is starting to wear off. Maybe once again I am feeling invincible, and think that waiting for tomorrow to take care of myself is OK.

Well, it's not OK, because tomorrow I will also be tired... and no stronger than I am today. So if I wait until tomorrow to eat healthier, then tomorrow I will have another reason to wait until the next day. And the next.

TODAY'S STATS

- 6 hours of sleep. (Boo.)
- 20 minutes of upper body work with the TRX Suspension Trainer and free weights at home after teaching a Spinning class.

Onward and forward.

Until tomorrow.

3

Dieter's Journal

DAY 3: EATING AT 2 A.M.

I guess I did not eat enough yesterday since I found myself awake at 2 a.m., searching for food. I settled for half of a protein bar, then went back to sleep. I usually don't wake up to eat, but obviously my body was looking for calories. I'm just lucky I did not have any chips around. I did make an effort to sleep last night, and slept in until 8:30 a.m. Felt a bit sluggish and tired this morning since I am not used to sleeping, but worked awhile, then exercised for 30 minutes. I started training with kettlebells again. I hate kettlebells. I really do. I love them, but I also despise them. Love/hate. Love/hate. Love/hate.

Kettlebells are the hardest thing I know, so I went easy on myself and did only two sets of double arm swings (x25), one set of single arm swings (x15 total), cursing out every number — 10 - f*!@ - 11 - sh*t - 12 - f!%@. To add insult to injury, I did one set of deep kettlebell squats.

So why do I work with kettlebells if I dislike them? Because they rock, they're effective, and I'm a glutton for punishment.

Kettlebells get your heart rate up and really tone your butt and thighs, which is why I took it easy with them today. I want to be able to sit (and teach Spinning) tomorrow. Knowing it was a "desk-day" and that I only had a limited amount

JOURNAL

of time to work out, I chose the kettlebells (along with my core work) to elevate my heart rate. Even if I don't have much time, I've found that I can always squeeze something short and intense into my day. When I work out I also tend to eat healthier.

NOT EATING ENOUGH

I was so absorbed in work that I really did not eat enough today. How do I know that? Because when I was at the grocery store I had to get a protein bar to eat in the car—I didn't think I would make it home without it. Of course I would have, but my brain was telling me I had to eat "now." I was able to pass the lovely little demons outside the store selling Girl Scout cookies. (*"Away demons! Away!"*) They were so cute and held out their tempting wares to corrupt me. I held my ground and continued into the store, where I was met with the smell of heavenly-scented French bread. Everywhere I went, something called my name, making me drool...and trying to get into my shopping cart.

If I had eaten enough earlier (or had even eaten a proper lunch), this trip to the store would not have been so painful. As I was putting away the groceries, I decided to get a spoon, and have a snippet of the frozen yogurt I had bought. It was the really good yogurt, too. Mmmm. It was all melty around the edges. The spoon just slipped and scooped so perfectly. Before I knew it, I'd scooped about 8 ounces into my mouth. I followed the yogurt with pickles (no, I am not pregnant—just weird).

Even though I ate breakfast this morning and had blueberries for a snack, by the time I hit the store at 4 p.m. I was famished...and you saw what happened then.

SAVING THE DAY

What does all this mean? Don't let yourself go hungry. It also means that I ate something light and healthy for dinner... something without sugar as this was a very "sugar heavy" day. On the bright side, I didn't use this slip as a "get out of jail free card" to start overeating. My total calories today will still be acceptable, though my food choices were not the best. I am trying, day-by-day, to improve my nutrition. There will be some back-sliding, but I'll get right back in the saddle. And by the way, never stand over a gallon of ice cream or yogurt with a spoon. Never. Just put some in a bowl and walk away when done.

TODAY'S STATS

- 8 hours of sleep (Huh?)
- 30 minutes of kettlebells and abdominal work.

Onward and forward.

Until tomorrow.

Dieter's Journal

4

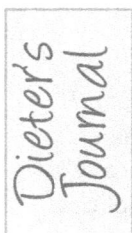

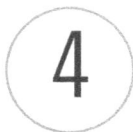

DAY 4: THE FAMINE IS COMING!

Right about now, days four through seven or so, your body is getting a clue as to what's going on. You are eating less and moving more. In nature, that means one thing: the famine is coming!

Your body holds onto fat for one reason—to get you through periods of starvation. What it doesn't realize is that there really is no famine...that there is plenty of food to go around (at least in our nation of excess). All it cares about is that you are depleting your stores of the very thing it counts on to keep you alive: fat. And now it's fighting back.

Today I am starving. Not literally starving, but the kind of starving where my body is sabotaging me. It's sending signals to my brain to trick me into eating. "*She's tired.*" "*She's hungry.*" "*She needs cookies.*" It's one of those collaborations that are deadly to our weight loss efforts.

This is where I need to stay focused and ask myself, "*Am I going to let my body win? Am I going to let my body's quest to keep the fat ruin my efforts?*" No, I will not.

Do you know why I won't give in? Because I have done this before. I know how this works. I know the feelings and pitfalls. And I also know that I can give in today, but if I start again tomorrow, in 4-5 days I'll be faced with the same situation: wanting to break down and eat a bunch of things that are physically not good for me (but mentally—mmm, yes). Just because my body said so.

> "My theory is this: take pain now or take it later. I'll take it now. It won't be any easier tomorrow. "

I was very tired this morning, but felt good during Spinning class. Afterward, I worked my upper body for about 30 minutes, this time at the gym so I could semi-goof off with my Spinning buds. Usually I weight train at home because, teaching at the gym as I do, I tend to stop what I am doing and interact with our members. As my friend Heather once told me, I am "Helpy Helperton." And being a Helperton doesn't get your workout done.

FEELING THE BULGE

A trick I used today to outsmart my body was to wear my smaller sweatpants around the house—the ones that used to be baggy on me. Feeling the fabric stretch over my, eh, assets helps keep me in line. It also reminds me that one of the reasons I am doing this is because I cannot afford a new, larger wardrobe. Necessity breeds action.

SHOCKINGLY...

One of the things I have been craving the last two days are pickles. I like all kinds of pickles, but the pickles I bought were the crunchy sweet whole ones. I checked the back of the jar by accident and discovered that each of these little pickles has 35 calories and 8 grams of sugar. I just ate six.

JOURNAL

In essence, I consumed 210 calories and 48 grams of sugar. Of *pickles*.

In contrast, my frozen yogurt has 120 calories and 14 grams of sugar per half cup. Even if I had eaten 8 ounces of the smooth chocolate-y wonder, I would actually be no worse off (and far more satisfied) than eating those measly six pickles.

So today's lesson? Never assume! I just blew my "fun" calories on cucumbers marinated in vinegar and sugar. How sad is that?

TODAY'S STATS

- 7 hours of sleep
- Taught an hour Spinning class plus performed 40 minutes of upper body weight training at gym
- 25 full push-ups (yes!)

Onward and forward.

Until tomorrow.

5

Dieter's Journal

DAY 5: 1 POUND UP

The Old Me Would Have Screamed!

Before I had my massive weight loss a few years back, if I had tried to lose weight and gained a pound it would have been the end of the world. I would eat every carbohydrate in sight, punishing myself for what I would perceive as something I had done wrong.

I weighed myself today, and I did not scream even though I weigh one pound more than when I started this project five days ago. Last time I lost between ¼ and ½ pound per day. Yes, I had a lot of weight to lose back then and yes, I was younger. But still...

Did I get discouraged?

No. I had a brief moment where I thought, "*Oh crap. All that work for nothing. What the...?*" Because I know that my weight fluctuates depending on how much salt I've eaten, where I am in my menstrual cycle, how much sleep I've gotten, and how much water I've ingested, I did not throw in the towel at this piece of bad news. I'm really not expecting any change in my weight for about two more weeks. That may be hard to swallow for some, considering all the "miraculous" results we see on television and read about in magazines,

JOURNAL

but it's the reality. There are many, many factors to consider when it comes to actual weight loss.

Just because I haven't lost anything measurable on a scale doesn't mean I'm not losing fat. Actual weight loss hinges on too many variables to hang our hats on one particular element. Fat loss, rather than weight loss, is something you can feel. Fat loss can be judged in terms of looks and clothing fit. Sometimes we need to say, "*To hell with the scale!*" and continue on. Could I have given up? Yes. But...

I look at it this way: I can either lose, maintain, or gain weight. The first two are OK. The third, not so much.

THE BENEFIT OF BEING UNFIT

I work out about 350 minutes per week on average. The "magic" number, according to the American College of Sports Medicine, is 250 minutes or more per week of exercise to speed up weight loss. (Read "*How Much Exercise Do You Need to Lose Weight?*" on page 144 if you haven't already.) However, when you already exercise a lot, your body gets accustomed to it and compensates accordingly. There is no "shock" to get your body going. For someone who hasn't exercised regularly, any type of physical activity is bound to kick-start weight loss, thus, someone who hasn't worked out at all but eats the same as I do will lose weight faster than I will. That's my reality.

SUGAR ALL THE WAY

I eat too much sugar and I know that already. Am I willing to give up the chocolate chips in my oatmeal I start each morning with? No, so I need to work around that. This story is about losing weight in the real world, where we are parents and spouses and employees or business owners. We don't have time to measure everything we put in our mouths. We are stressed, busy, and tired, but we can still make adjustments that benefit our health and help us reach our goals. It might just take a little bit longer.

Based on what I've written this week, the adjustments I need to make to spur my weight loss are:

- Sleep more
- Eat less sugar
- Drink more water
- Make sure I eat before I head out
- Eat more fruits and vegetables
- Add something different to my exercise program

This is what I will be implementing next week. It's all about fine-tuning what works for our own bodies. No two people are alike, and not all solutions work for everyone. We make a change, monitor the result, and tweak. Make a change, monitor the result, and tweak.

NEAR EATING

I wasn't even hungry today, so why was I fantasizing about a carb-laden binge? Because I slept less than five hours last night and when I am tired, I eat. I had low-fat frozen yogurt again earlier when I couldn't stay awake. Not a deal-breaker but not the best of choices. It's all about making better and better choices, every meal, every day.

I tell you, though, if I were not writing this series I would probably be eating. Now I feel naked and accountable to

JOURNAL

people I can't even see. It's weird, but effective too, I suppose. I thought of sneaking in some snacks and not documenting it, but then I realized how pointless that would be. If I am going to eat, I am going to tell you. Why? Because I am not perfect. Why pretend that weight loss is easy? The road to hell is paved with good intentions.

> *If I lie to you, I am helping no one. I have fitness pro friends who lie to their students and clients. They lie about what they eat. They lie about being balanced. They pretend to be perfect and happy, admired for their amazing bodies, all while secretly binging and then vomiting up their food in the bathroom. It's so sad to see. Lies, lies, lies. I don't do lies. Lies set everyone up for failure.*

TODAY'S STATS

- 4.5 hours of sleep
- 30 hard, consistent minutes of stomach and back training, butt workout, and kettlebells. One set of double-arm kettlebell swings (x25 f*&!), two sets single-arm kettlebell swings (x20 f*&!), two sets of deep kettlebell squats (x8 f*&! + f*&!).

Onward and forward.

Until tomorrow.

6

Dieter's Journal

DAY 6: CLOUDY WEATHER SNACK-A-THON

Cloudy days and cold weather always inspire me to eat. I think it's a "hibernation" thing. Today, I just wanted to eat, snuggle under the covers, and sleep all day.

To counteract doing something detrimental to my progress I made sure that I ate every two hours or so, tricking myself into thinking I was snacking.

After breakfast and teaching a Spinning class, I had a small sugar-free vanilla latte with soy milk, then an hour later ordered a warm and filling Chinese vegetable dish that had tofu and brown rice.

I ate only ⅓ of the meal at lunch because I wasn't very hungry (the coffee had filled me up). Throughout the day, I snacked on the remainder of the food, in about ⅓ increments. This helped me feel constantly full, feel like I was eating a lot—fulfilling my desire to snack—and still kept me within a reasonable daily calorie count. It gave me a nice serving of vegetables and fiber, too.

It's good sometimes to "fake yourself out." The constant small eating helped me feel like I was eating a lot, and it was just what the dreary day ordered.

JOURNAL

STIFF AND SORE — OH YAY

I'm a little stiff and sore today. Yesterday's kettlebells fried my thighs and butt, and since I challenged my core a bit more my abdominals were tender, an area usually hard for me to target. My shoulders are feeling the workout I did at the gym after class. I used mostly free weights today, with a "pyramid up" structure, i.e. starting with a lower weight set first, mid-weight second set, and heavier weight on the last set. Then I played with a pulley cable machine and decided I liked the pulleys and the way the cables move with me, yet independent of each other. Though I prefer bodyweight, kettlebells and free weights, I like machines that work like the human body does, and doesn't "lock you into" a particular position. The more variety in workouts the better, I say. Keeps my body on its toes.

FEELING STRONGER

I was definitely feeling stronger mentally and physically today. That urge to overeat is actually gone. I'm surprised this early in the game. But it will come back again. This I know. It's all about outlasting and outsmarting cravings.

TODAY'S STATS

- 6.5 hours of sleep
- 1-hour Spinning class, followed by 30 minutes of upper body weight training at the gym

Onward and forward.

Until tomorrow.

7

Dieter's Journal

DAY 7: REST

One day a week I take a complete break from exercise. No Spinning, no strength training, not even any stretching. It's one day for my body to go, "*Ahhhhh*," and just kick back. Usually this day is Sunday.

A few years ago, when I was at my fittest, things were different. I used to get up early and ride my bike on Sundays. In the summer my friends and I would meet at 6 a.m. before it got hot (and while the kids were sleeping) and take long, strenuous rides. We'd push mile after mile, hill after hill, challenge after challenge, returning home exhausted and sweaty to prepare breakfast for our families as they began to stir. In the winter we'd head out with long cycling tights, gloves, and windbreakers, cold and miserable the whole way.

An early, very chilly morning (an Easter Sunday, in fact), I got stuck returning down the side of a mountain that I'd ridden up. It was raining, freezing, and we had ice in our hair. No one else was on the road, we had no cell phone reception, and my friend and I had to pull off to the side, shivering uncontrollably, wondering if we'd ever make it down alive. Another Sunday morning I was following a group of experienced cyclists through some canyons. They were far ahead of me, out of sight, and I was trying to catch up. I put everything I had into each pedal stroke, and barreled

JOURNAL

over the crest, missing my turn and almost toppling off the cliff. Those were my Sundays.

One day, while getting ready to head out on a cold early-morning Sunday ride by myself, I discovered I had a flat tire. I looked at the tire. Pondered. Then I removed my cycling gear, headed back upstairs, and jumped into my warm, toasty bed. I haven't gotten up early to ride on a Sunday since.

Now every Sunday morning is "quiet time." I drink warm tea, take my time with breakfast, and read a book or watch the news for a few minutes. It's the one day where we don't have to rush, and the day I usually don't exercise.

Rest days are important to keep us working hard. I lost track of that and wore myself out by not allowing rest days . Just like when performing intervals, we can't give 100% if we don't know when our recoveries (rest days) are. And we stop enjoying what we do.

CRITICAL MASS

Scheduled days of rest also give you a chance to renew your motivation. Continuous exercise can wear you down and wear you out. You stop working as hard, start cutting your workout time, stop lifting as heavy, or running as far. What once was a passion has now become just a chore that you dread. Why? Because you didn't allow yourself rest time... time to physically and mentally recover. Having that one day to look forward to as an exercise "rest day" allows you to work harder during the week and keeps you focused.

Don't believe me? Try it. While most people are looking for excuses not to work out, if you are exercising regularly, look at your calendar and pencil in a specific day where you do not work out at all. Write it down. Make it part of your schedule. You may find you are more motivated with your workouts, knowing that you are drawing closer and closer to your "rest day." Again, it's "faking yourself out." You might be more willing to try a new class or perform an extra set of push-ups, safe in the knowledge that your recovery is on the horizon.

BALANCING ACT

It took me two years to get to this point where exercise is good again and I am not dreading it. I am even considering starting to ride my bike on the open road again (I stopped after the "near-cliff" experience). I enjoy Spinning once more, and I really savor my day of rest. Sometimes, when I am busy, deadlines force an unscheduled day of rest during the workweek and I am OK with that, too.

It's all about balance now. Balancing exercise, food, and life. No excesses (except the work part. I am still working on that). Give yourself that day off...and find your balance.

TODAY'S STATS

- 7 hours of sleep
- No exercise. Day of rest.

Onward and forward.

Until tomorrow.

Dieter's Journal

8

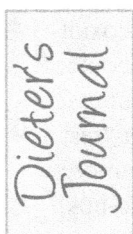

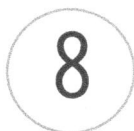

DAY 8: ANTICIPATE

My day of rest yesterday was much needed because this week
I have a challenging first few days: teaching two Spinning
classes today and one tomorrow morning. That's three hard
Spinning classes in 24 hours. For me, this is difficult because
I give 100% in each class, and there's not much time to re-
charge in between. I usually don't teach "2-in-a-day" classes
because it is pointless to exercise that much, and if I do that
too often I stop enjoying it. Right now I still enjoy teaching.

PLAN FOR TEMPTATION

Anticipating what's coming up in my week exercise-wise,
work-wise, stress-wise, and event-wise is a way for me to
keep on track. If I am going somewhere where I will be
tempted with delicious but calorie-dense foods, I can "calorie-
down" a few days before, which will allow me my inevitable
slip into momentary bliss without the onslaught of guilt. I
may be determined, but I am human, after all, and have a
hard time keeping my hand out of a cookie jar.

Thinking about what is coming up also allows me to schedule
more days of rest if I will need them, or more weight training if I have been teaching too many cardio classes. Today I
knew there would be nothing more than some brief abdominal
exercises in terms of strength training. My body needed all

of its available energy to pull through those classes without tearing myself down. Again, it's about balance. I no longer exercise compulsively on certain days because I think I have to—even though I am PMS bloated like today. I have learned to be flexible and to listen to my body, not the voices in my head. Anticipating my week helps me keep a sense of balance.

TODAY'S STATS

- 7 hours of sleep.
- Taught two strength-style Spinning classes (lots of hills—yay); 15 minutes of abdominals.

Onward and forward.

Until tomorrow.

Dieter's Journal

9

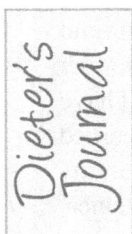

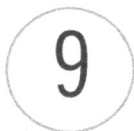

DAY 9: EXHAUSTION

When well-laid out plans go awry, you just hang on to the seat of your cycling shorts and try for the best. This is a short day by my wordy standards.

A day that started with a sick child who was up half the night (and mommy with her), a Spinning class, and deadlines for design clients ended with an evening business event, homework fights, dinner, and then—collapse and cry. Even a superwoman has her limits.

It took all I had today to stay on track. I ate a little too much, but overall it's not a deal breaker. I was proud of myself for that. I ate some low-fat yogurt after dinner for recharging. Then I made an executive decision: no more work tonight. Get the kids ready for bed and hit the sack.

Sometimes we need to recognize our limits...and respect them. I could have consoled myself with overeating, like the "old me" used to do. Sometimes the weight on my shoulders can momentarily be lightened by heavenly brownies. Instead, today I focused on getting through the day hour-by-hour, project-by-project. A few extra carbs kept me going. Compromise is what keeps me sane now.

Advice: exhaustion. Don't let yourself go there.

TODAY'S STATS

- 7 hours of sleep
- Taught one Spinning class, did no weight training.

Onward and forward.

Until tomorrow.

Dieter's Journal

(10)

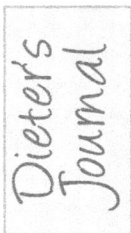

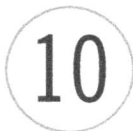

DAY 10: CRAVING CARBS

I've never tasted Miracle Whip® until today.

My daughter asked me to buy it on our last shopping trip, and as I was making her a sandwich I wiped the knife with my finger and had a taste. It was pretty good. This was the light kind, mind you, so it only had 1.5 grams of fat per serving. I had no reason to eat it since it wasn't lunch time but I bet would have tasted great on bread topped with provolone cheese.

Sweet, salt, or...carbs?

I think it's the saltiness that drew me to the Miracle Whip. I've been thinking about salt all day. I had three potato chips in the car and I've been thinking about popcorn for some reason. I even ate a few dill pickles. (I learned my lesson with those higher calorie sweet pickles.)

I am keeping my eye on the final prize (fitting into my jeans that are now about 3" from closing — 3" might as well be 3' as far as those pants go).

My eating is slipping a little bit again. Not so much in terms of binging (I am no longer polishing off a batch of cookies), but overall I am eating more and more carbs, more and more frequently. This definitely has something to do with my monthly cycle.

The question is, how do I pull back on carbs without becoming tired? How do I eat more fruit and veggies, for example, when what I really crave are breads? I need a certain amount of carbs to keep up with my Spinning schedule. I can't run out of energy when I teach. It's one thing to peter out on the bike when you are the student—it's a whole other thing to peter out when you are leading an entire class. But I know the sugars stored in my muscles will get me through most anything, which is why I start most mornings with oatmeal or protein pancakes.

Overall, I am a believer in eating carbs. I lost more than 80 pounds in the past consuming them. The trick is to eat more of the good kind, less of the refined. The trick is to find the balance between what works for weight loss and having a life. As always, that's the most complicated part of the puzzle. If I was promised an eternal size 4 in exchange for giving up carbs forever I would say, *"Never mind."*

As Rule #32 from the movie Zombieland states, *"Enjoy the Little Things."* I enjoy my little carbs...but maybe I should just enjoy fewer of them?

TODAY'S STATS

- 6 hours of sleep
- No exercise! (Unplanned day of rest because client deadlines and sick children got the best of me.)

Onward and forward.

Until tomorrow.

Dieter's Journal (11)

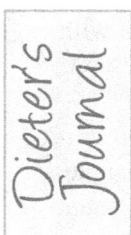

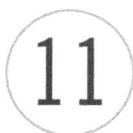

DAY 11: FITTING IT IN

Todaywasabusydaylamgoingtogofast.

Whew! When your day is very busy it's hard to stick with your goals. Deadlines, sick kids, stress, and life in general can take a toll on your most well-laid plans.

Today I was very busy with both children home from school. I needed to sub out my Spinnning class, much to my dismay and sadness. I tried to stay with healthy eating but remembered only one fruit and a wilted spinach salad.

I did a briefer-than-brief upper body workout today followed by 10 minutes of punching a boxing bag. That was all I could muster before sitting back down at my desk.

Why bother with so little, you ask? Because anything is better than nothing. Seriously. 15–20 minutes of intense, concentrated work can trump an hour-long session if you do it right. More than anything, though, any kind of exercise is good for you mentally.

There are few basic "checklist" items to I try to stick with when busy:
• Drink lots of water
• Eat a vegetable "to go"

- Eat some protein
- Give yourself one healthy-ish treat

If you can remember just those few simple things you should be able to get through the day without completely sabotaging yourself.

NOBODY'S PERFECT

Not to mean that I was perfect—in fact, today was a less than stellar day nutritionally. I had four handfuls of a cereal/cracker mix somewhere in there, which was an unsatisfactory waste of calories. It's way too easy to grab an unhealthy snack in a busy day.

One apple and that spinach and tomato salad were my only fruits and veggies. I really need to focus on the "5-a-day" or more (the 9-a-day is far out of my league). Somewhere between the carbs and the dairy I am faltering with what is most important....what comes directly from the earth.

Other than the snack mix, I made a coffee smoothie concoction to keep me awake: coffee, stevia, nonfat milk blended with nonfat frozen yogurt. It was my treat, filling, and kept me going. (I've learned since to add protein powder to the mix and suddenly this beverage is a lot healthier!)

THE WORKOUT, OR LACK THEREOF

I am starting to feel out of sorts since I have not taught a Spinning class since Tuesday morning and I will not be back on the bike until Saturday. That's pure misery for an indoor cycling lover like me. Spinning classes not only burn calories and keep my cardiovascular system in great shape, but it helps with my head as well. Hard cardiovascular exercise releases much-needed endorphins—one of our pain killing hormones—and seems to clear the cobwebs to allow for clearer thinking.

While I did not release much in the way of endorphins, I performed a brief bout of strength training. I moved from exercise to exercise, with no rest, working hard and steady. That was all I had time for, but I was able hit everything in my upper body in record time.

There probably were no strength gains today, but the goal was no strength losses. Whenever we go on any kind of "diet" (and I use that term loosely), we lose muscle along with fat.

My goal is to try to maintain what I have for muscle and lose some of what I have of fat.

TODAY'S STATS

- 6.5 hours of sleep
- Upper body workout

Onward and forward.

Until tomorrow.

(END) *Dieter's Journal*

DAYS 12/13: FINALLY LOSING WEIGHT

I got on the scale this morning I was down 1.5 pounds. Finally!

I had a few food challenges to overcome today: pizza with family members and then a trip to the movies, which meant popcorn. Movie theater popcorn is very, very high in calories and fat. The Center for Science in the Public Interest found that a Regal Theater medium popcorn, about 20 cups, contains 1,200 calories and 60 grams of saturated fat. So although I had maybe 1/3 of a medium popcorn (sneaking handfuls from the kids), I am still looking at 400 calories and 20 grams of fat—for a snack. Plus the pizza and brownie. My total calories today were probably around 2,000—not low enough for weight loss but not enough to gain, considering I burned at least 500 calories at the gym this morning. It's so hard to burn calories and so very easy to pack 'em in.

Eating more today means that tomorrow will be a lighter day to compensate.

Onward and forward.

The end.

Food/Exercise Tracker

Keeping track
keeps you on track.

FOOD LOG

DATE: _____

FOOD	PROTEIN (GRAMS)	CARB (GRAMS)	FAT (GRAMS)	CALORIES
MEAL _____				
Time _____				
_____ _____				
_____				
SNACK_____				
Time _____				
_____ _____				
_____				
MEAL _____				
Time _____				
_____ _____				
_____				
SNACK_____				
Time _____				
_____ _____				
_____				
MEAL _____				
Time _____				
_____ _____				
_____				
SNACK_____				
Time _____				
_____ _____				
_____				
DAILY TOTAL				

WATER: ☐ ☐ ☐ ☐ ☐ ☐ ☐ ☐

VEGGIES: ☐ ☐ ☐ ☐ ☐   (check off your total servings each day and try to fill all the boxes)

EXERCISE LOG

	CARDIO	STRENGTH	FLEXIBILITY
DAY 1 Minutes Type			
DAY 2 Minutes Type			
DAY 3 Minutes Type			
DAY 4 Minutes Type			
DAY 5 Minutes Type			
DAY 6 Minutes Type			
WEEKLY GOAL			
ACTUAL TOTAL			

(download PDF files of both forms at
www.realworldweightloss.com/21daysbook)

"That's a Wrap"

"The human body is the only
machine for which there are
no spare parts."

~Hermann M. Biggs

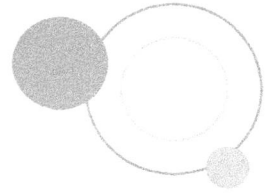

"So Long, Farewell, Auf Wiedersehen, Adieu"

"It's gettin' it's gettin' it's gettin' kinda heavy. I've got the power."
~Snap

You find yourself sitting there, a box of cookies in your lap, an empty bag of chips at your feet, a gallon of ice cream half gone. And you wonder, *"What happened to my desire to lose weight? What happened to me?"*

You might ask yourself where you went wrong, why you cracked, or how you ended up on this eating binge. *"Why didn't I say no?"* you question. *"Why couldn't I just walk away? Why wasn't I stronger?"*

The reason, simply and honestly, is that you didn't want to be strong...because perhaps you no longer believe in your own strength.

Sometimes we let life beat us down. Our day-to-day activities take away much of what is intrinsically "us" at the core. It is our core that is vibrant, strong, healthy, full of life, love, and passion. Sometimes our core beings get buried, though, and we forget who we are, and mostly—how strong we are. We somehow need to reconnect to what is "us" and find the power inside to change.

Take a moment to look back at your life. Think of all the things you *did* do. Maybe you've survived a serious childhood illness, lost a beloved pet, overcome your first heartbreak, aced a test you thought you'd fail, or finished college while working full-time. Maybe you've experienced a firing or a layoff, given birth, gone through an ugly divorce, lost a parent or a spouse, received an unexpected promotion, walked away from a car accident, or found your soul mate. Possibly you've excelled at a sport, learned a new hobby, survived a surgery, or cried with happiness at your child's graduation.

> " Grab those little moments and reflect on your loves and losses "

Make a list of what you've overcome and what you've accomplished. Then look at the cookies—directly into their beady, evil (yummy) chocolate chip eyes—and ask yourself, *"I did all of that and I can't do this? I can't say 'no, not right now?' I can't lose weight? Really? I can!"*

Answer that question to yourself. If you can remember the feelings of empowerment or the relief after surviving something traumatic you will realize that you can say no...that you really are as strong and capable now as you were then.

And you've got the power again, baby. I'll see you on the "thinner" side.

~Helen

CONNECT WITH ME!

Blog: www.realworldweightloss.com

Twitter: aspinchick

Facebook:
realworldweightloss
helenmryanfb

Pinterest: helenmryan

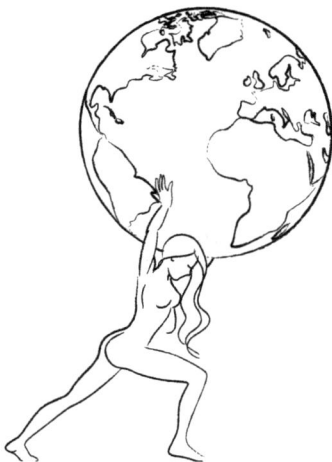

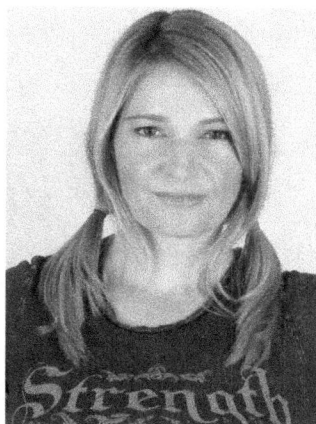

Helen Ryan is a freelance writer, speaker, and "life reinventor."

Ryan overcame her own challenges with weight and lost 82 pounds. She became a fitness pro to help others lose weight, get healthy and change their lives. Ryan is an ACE-certified personal trainer, certified Pilates instructor and certified Spinning® instructor.

In her free time, Ryan interviews rock stars, photographs rock concerts, and eats chocolate (really). She still teaches Spinning classes, which is her passion—and one of the things that saved her life. Ryan lives in California, and has two children.

DID YOU KNOW?

One of the best ways to feel better about yourself is to help others. Find a cause that means something to you and simply help out. The cause close to my heart? Domestic violence. I focus my energy helping our local domestic violence resource agency. *Do something good for someone else...and you'll reap the rewards.*

Web site: www.21daystochangeyourbody.com
(to access bonus content, use reference code 911)

www.ingramcontent.com/pod-product-compliance
Lightning Source LLC
Chambersburg PA
CBHW060452280326
41933CB00014B/2733